Sheldon Mindfulness
Keeping a Journal

Philip Cowell is an author, copywriter and poet. He has an eclectic mindfulness background and has participated in the Mindfulness-Based Stress Reduction course and other mindfulness-related training, including Focusing, Hakomi, Feldenkrais, Sacred Clown, and Courage and Renewal. He teaches creative writing in different settings and integrates mindfulness into his workshops. <www.philipcowell.co.uk>

D0528690

Sheldon Mindfulness

Selected titles

A full list of titles is available from Sheldon Press,
36 Causton Street, London SW1P 4ST and on our website at
www.sheldonpress.co.uk

Sheldon Mindfulness

Keeping a Journal

PHILIP COWELL

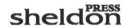
sheldon PRESS

First published in Great Britain in 2016

Sheldon Press
36 Causton Street
London SW1P 4ST
www.sheldonpress.co.uk

British Library Cataloguing-in-Publication Data
A catalogue record for this book is available from the British Library

ISBN 978-1-84709-378-3
eBook ISBN 978-1-84709-379-0

Typeset by Fakenham Prepress Solutions, Fakenham, Norfolk NR21 8NN
First printed in Great Britain by Ashford Colour Press
Subsequently digitally reprinted in Great Britain

eBook by Fakenham Prepress Solutions, Fakenham, Norfolk NR21 8NN

Produced on paper from sustainable forests

For my amazing parents, Sue and David Cowell,
who taught me how to love reading and writing

Contents

Acknowledgements

Thank you to Fiona Marshall at Sheldon Press for inviting me to write this book. You're a gift of an editor, being kind, thoughtful and grounding all at once.

Thank you to all the amazing mindfulness teachers out there. You do amazing work, and thanks especially to my own: Bangor University-trained Lorraine Millard – you're my guru through and through.

Thank you to all my amazing friends for nudging me along and inspiring me in so many ways – a special call out to John Biggin, Retta Bowen, Tamsin Clark, Julia Forster, Cate Hall, Susanna Howard, Ariane Koek, Kim Patrick, Anna Selby, Sarah Sheldon and Simon Timblick. And thank you Matt Anderson, my partner in life and laughter, for putting up with all the tapping away I did at our table, and for taking me to the movies. Love you all.

On my way to finishing this book, our green and blue planet lost one of its finest stewards, and one of my mum's dearest friends: Mary Cline. Mary embodied mindfulness in everything she did and her passions and loving-kindness live on through her gorgeous grown-up children. She was simply, unutterably, wonderful.

1

Calling all investigative journalists of the heart

You only have moments to write

Moments are all there is. Like this moment, the one you're reading this sentence in.

Each moment is a party invitation. It is either an invitation to be in the moment of the party we call life, or it is an invitation to write or speak or wriggle or do something else in the moment. Either way, the key is to turn up to whatever it is, with a half-smile, a party-popper in your pocket and a big homemade banner that says WELCOME.

Start writing right now

Five sentences. They don't have to be amazing sentences: just five sentences that somehow talk to you in this moment. They could just be five one-word sentences, or five 100-word sentences, whatever you want. Perhaps they sum up how you're feeling right now; perhaps you'll describe what you're wearing, where you're sitting, how you found this book, where you are in your life in this minute. You could even welcome five things that are here. Whatever five sentences you write, however rubbish or brilliant you're feeling, just do it. Then it's done, isn't it? You could keep them or throw them away, or post them to a friend, or plonk them on the compost. Do whatever is easy for you in this moment.

When you consider mindfulness, in whatever form it takes, you're essentially welcoming yourself *to* yourself. And welcome's a good word here: after all, it ends in 'me'. So hats off and welcome to this book, to you, to me, to *your* me, the me in you that lives, whose heart beats and who writes or wants to write. Welcome.

There are three things to do when mindful journalling

Mindful journalling is a mindfulness-inspired self-study practice that involves three very simple things, which – like any mindfulness practice – require practice, practice, practice. Here are the three ways to journal mindfully:

1 *First you gather – prepare to journal* How you do this is up to you. I'll give you some ideas in Chapter 3. The key is to notice that you're about to write; you're about to be writing; you're about to *be* the writing. Bring attention to coming to journal. Noticing your breathing is good for starters. I call this first stage Gathering; it's a bit like gathering up the bottom of your big dress before you plonk yourself down.

2 *Then you jot – write, with kind attention* This is Chapter 4. With mindful journalling, we write, knowing we are writing. We might use the physicality of the hand shifting across the page to bring us back to our attentiveness, just as mindful meditators use the breath as a focal point of theirs. The writing itself brings the writing into focus and awareness. We might write about the details of the day which are also the details of our awareness or mindfulness: the feel of the weather, that small smile you exchanged with a stranger, how underneath a bit of anger you felt some tiredness. I call this second stage Jotting – the plain, physical act of writing in cahoots with a kind, curious mind that's simply up for noticing. I use the word 'jotting' in particular because its etymology is useful for us here: coming from the Greek word *iota* for the letter 'i' – jotting is about the 'I' that writes, your I/eye. When it comes to any mindfulness practice, the question 'Who am I?' is never

far away. So the I jots itself down. In Chapter 4, I've prepared for you 31 mindful journal writing exercises – one for each day of the month – so you can have a go right away.

3 *Finally you wonder – pause and reflect* This is Chapter 5. Reflecting needn't be anything too intense. So you pause, noticing you're pausing, and reflect on what you've just done. This can be very quick or you can spend longer on it (you choose what's right for you). You might even find you reflect so much that you head back (or body back, perhaps) into journalling – first Gathering yourself, then Jotting away again. It's fine to keep scribbling, as long as you always leave the process through Wondering, allowing the possibility for a little pause, before you carry forward with your life.

So mindful journal practice, then: Gathering, Jotting, Wondering

The whole three-part process could take five minutes, or a whole day. It's really easy and difficult at once and I highly recommend it to you.

Mindful journalling is like wild swimming

Another name for mindful journalling, or mindful journal practice, might be wild journalling. Keeping a regular diary: that's like going to a swimming pool in order to keep fit. It's essential, don't get me wrong; we need a place to jot down our activities, our to-do list, plans for birthdays, perhaps the odd description of what happened. But when we take off out into the wilderness and swim naked in lakes and seas, we leave the everydayness of regular swimming behind. We plunge into the darkness and the murkiness. We see adventure rather than timetable, waterfalls rather than showers. Wild journalling is what happens when we exchange the swimming pool for the lagoon: the to-do list for simply to-be.

I am excited about you starting your own heart book

You'll fill it with multidimensional notes about sensations in the body and emotional weather states, thoughts about ideas and ideas about thoughts, descriptions of the sensing of your physical self, snippets captured from overheard conversations on buses, felt senses written in felt tip, confessions and imaginations, quotes from your favourite writers, lines of poems to be written and poems that have been written. After all, a mindful journal is all these things and more:

- Sometimes, a mindful journal entry is a description of what it's like looking out of the window in this moment, your feet firmly on the floor.
- Sometimes, it's an ambition written down for a future world, a hope for a kinder planet, a resolution to renew, your awareness always rooted in your body.
- Sometimes, it's a stepping out of the light and into the shadow, a reflection on a sadness, or a shame, or a past – or continuing – pain and its bodily ramifications for you in this moment.
- Sometimes, it's a reflection on relationships with people, institutions, abstract concepts and how these settle with you in the here and now.
- Sometimes, the mindful journal entry is just 'concerned with language on a very plain level', as John Ashbery writes in his poem 'Paradoxes and Oxymorons': plain language trying to capture plain experience, right here, right now.

Secular mindfulness + journal writing = mindful journal practice

A mindful journal is a book where, to adapt Jon Kabat-Zinn's definition of mindfulness, you pay attention in a particular way, on purpose, in the present moment, non-judgementally, through writing:

- You could write a mindful journal entry about something that happened earlier in the week: the difference between that and a normal journal entry is that you'd probably be writing about the past event with powerful reference to your continuing present felt experience.

- You could write a mindful journal entry about the present moment, in this moment, describing the feel of your hand across the page, the beating of your pulse, the way the clouds slowly move outside the window as you write.
- You could write a mindful journal entry about the future, where you consolidate plans and sketch out a dream, all the time with your feet firmly planted on the floor, your future plans intermingled with descriptions of bodily sensations in the present moment.

With mindful journal practice, we intend to write and write to intend

A mindful journal involves an intention to write, knowing you are writing. We might distinguish the mindful journal from the allegedly ordinary journal, or the unmindful journal, or even the mindless journal. With wild journalling, you're writing knowing you are writing. Perhaps it's even less personal than that: writing knowing the writing. Can we even shorten it (and perhaps we'll whisper it under our breath from time to time as we keep our mindful journals)? *Writing, knowing.*

In this sense, the mindful journal act – that specific act of writing down an entry in your mindful journal – is itself another opportunity to experiment how to live a full and wonderful life, no matter what pleasures or pains we experience in this moment. The writing act itself – if it slips into the realm of gentle, detached observation – becomes another form of mindfulness meditation, a laboratory we can step into to start our new experiments for living. The writing itself becomes another meditation practice, or dignity, like sitting practice or mindful standing or walking. We could call it journal meditation.

A mindful journal could be a notebook, a diary, a bunch of blank pages, a blog . . .

Perhaps the pages are blank or have lines. It might be a notebook that's part of your favourite kind of stationery, or perhaps like me you don't care too much how it looks. As long as we bring awareness even to this act of taking our paper – approaching the page – in the same way we'd bring attention to the act of taking our seat in sitting meditation.

Your journal might not even be in one place at all. That works for me. You might consider anywhere where you jot down your mindful words to be your journal, pasted over various of the transitional surfaces of our lives: a Post-it™ note here, an online status update there, the back of your hand, marginalia in a novel you're reading, the poster you annotate in that public space. You might even consider the whole world your journal and you are walking through it, writing on its various sheets and platforms. To what extent are you up for being a mindful graffiti artist of the heart?

You'll find your own mindful journal practice

There are loads of ways of keeping a mindful journal practice and the key thing is to find your own authentic way, rooted in what works for you:

- Emily Dickinson wrote poems on the back of envelopes and stuffed them into her desk drawers. You could say that was her mindful journal practice.
- The poet Frank O'Hara would walk out into the streets of New York City on his lunch break and type whole complete poems on typewriters in shops. You could say that was part of his mindful journal practice.
- The Burmese poet and comedian Zargana, sentenced to 59 years' imprisonment in 2008 for criticizing the generals (he was released in 2013), wrote poems with his fingers in the dust of his prison cell floor. That was his mindful journal practice.

You'll find your own patterns of writing and habits of keeping a mindful journal, your own notebooks, envelopes, typewriters and floors to write on. After all, that's half of the work, isn't it, noticing your patterns and habits, where the pen or the pencil falls (if it does at all). This work is all about bringing yourself back to the present moment through writing: writing with intention and attention. Writing, knowing. *Writing knowingly.*

Mindful journalling *is* lifelong learning

Keeping a mindful journal is about you saying yes to life and to your learning adventures within it. The party-popper in your pocket – that symbol of the potential for celebration at any moment – is never far away. We'll talk more about learning in a bit, but if you keep a mindful journal – if you write from your body and your breath, with all your heart – you will learn new things about yourself, the world and your relationship with it.

Mindful journal practice is a form of mindfulness-inspired self-study

You will walk around the habitat of your habits and spot traits you hadn't noticed before; you'll have 'Ah-ha!' moments when you find long-term, overarching patterns in yourself that you wouldn't have spotted otherwise. You will learn facts – concrete facts – about your lived experience, and that includes the highs as well as the lows. You will become an expert in your own equanimity; each of your entries will become small lectures that contribute to your Master's in loving-kindness. It's a fascinating area because you are both student and lecturer in this night class about the day. You are both imparting knowledge and taking it in – and here it's less knowledge, more knowing. With this work, you are teaching yourself how to learn from yourself; you're learning how to learn and teach at the same time.

I see mindful journal writing as a kind of gentle rocking and rolling

Mindful journal practice is a kind of awakening and self-nourishing through words and kindness in the here and now. If a famous poet like Emily Dickinson writes on the back of an envelope, or if we scribble a mindful journal entry into our big notepad, we're all doing the same thing by my book: we're engaging in the 'one wild and precious' (Mary Oliver) act of transcribing our lives, saying, 'Yes, yes, *yes*' to possibility with our whole bodies, treading out (with big boots) into the landscape of our sovereign selves.

Journalling is really, really popular (let's do it mindfully)

And it doesn't look as if the popularity will wane very soon (and nor should it, of course). Just look at Facebook and Twitter and other social media platforms to see what I mean – they're all kinds of journal keeping (not necessarily mindful, of course). Capturing the variety and quality of lived experience has as much to do with keeping a journal as it does keeping a Facebook wall. OK, with Facebook we're writing with an audience in mind, aren't we (are we?), but perhaps we're doing the same even in the privacy of a diary under lock and key:

- Who do we have in mind when we're writing our journal?
- Who do we have in body when we're writing our journal?
- Who is with us as we write?
- Who do we write our journal for?
- Who is doing the writing?

These are all really good questions, and probably useful questions if you're embarking on the work of the heart in written form, as it seems you are, you lovely person.

We're getting somewhere and we're not getting somewhere

There is nowhere else we need to be but here. It's here, the answer is here. It's here in you, right now. Just begin. Start writing your mindful journal. You know how to do it already.

Write right away

Find your journal (whether it's a regular notebook or one of many different kinds of journal surfaces we've already talked about) and just write. It's as simple as that. Write whatever comes to mind and body, for as long as you like. Just write. Don't worry about it. Write. I know we've already done that but it's just good to write, and you already know how to write, so come, welcome, write.

How was that?

How does it feel now, having written what you've just written? What is here in the aftermath of what you have just done? And maybe you didn't write. Maybe it's just nice to think about writing, or enough to know you will do a little writing later. We might say to ourselves, 'I'll do some writing in time.' There's no rush with mindful journal practice. You can't push the river, as the Buddhists say.

Practise sitting down

As writers, sitting down is something we're really good at. Perhaps we're too good at it! If you're sitting down right now, do you remember how you did it? Did you rush into your seat, perhaps, without thinking (I know I did) or did you manage to slow down and realize which foot went first in that great tangling game we call sitting? Given we're going to be sitting down a lot over the course of reading this book and writing your journal, why not practise bringing kind attention to the simple act of taking your seat?

Here's how. Stand up and sit down a few times. Vary the speed. Include a little walk up to your seat, if you like. Change the way you sit down, the angle, what you attend to with your senses. Pour weight into your left side, then your right side. What's different? Experiment with your own variations. Bring attention to your contact with the seat. Imagine you're sitting right in the middle of your life. What does it feel like? If you fancy it, start writing about 'sittingdownness' in your journal (you're likely to be sitting down, but why not write first standing up?). Write a piece called 'How I sat down like this' or 'An ode to my chair' or 'Ten ways of sitting down', or just start writing without a title for eight minutes about your experience of taking your seat. How much giving is involved in taking your seat? Who sits? Is a feeling of gratitude possible here? When you sit down, does your breath sit down too?

Mindfulness is paying attention in a particular way, on purpose

We'll talk more about mindfulness in Chapter 2, and the chances are you know a lot about it already. Being with present, moment-to-moment experience, as it unfolds here and now, and observing it all with kindness and gentleness, without judgement, observing thoughts without following them – that's something like mindfulness. I say 'something like' because it's really important you find your own words for defining mindfulness. Finding your own account of mindfulness is part of the work of keeping a mindful journal. That handsome essayist, Emerson, invited his readers to write their own Bibles, so I too invite you to define your own mindfulness through practice, practice, practice.

Mindfulness is both thousands of years old and relatively new

It's thousands of years old because mindfulness was one of the fundamental teachings of the Buddha; it's relatively new because it's only been in the last 35 years or so that pioneers like Jon Kabat-Zinn, Mark Williams, Rebecca Crane and Sarah Silverton have shown us the efficacy of mindfulness for stress reduction, depression and coping with illness.

Mindfulness is both a training in attention and awareness – a set of skills you can learn – and an overall approach to life that involves befriending yourself through simple and continuing embodied self-awareness. So it's about:

- sitting, and being the knowing you are sitting;
- when standing, really standing;
- walking in beauty;
- writing and knowing (non-conceptually) the writing, as we'll practise with mindful journalling.

Bring attention to your hands

Writers, like other creative practitioners, use their hands a lot. Whether you write with a pen or type like a trooper, your hands are precious and deserve nurturing as much as any bit of you. Nurturing here can be using your favourite hand cream, but also bringing simple awareness to your hands. Here are some ideas to warm up before journalling. It's a bit like holding your hands while you take them for a walk:

1 Hold your hands together in whatever way feels natural. Bring wonder to them: are you clasping, grasping, cradling, rubbing? What words best describe your kind of hand holding?
2 Can you shake your own hands?
3 Rub your palms together as if you're warming them by a fire. Do this gently and quickly – and with a bit of speed – for ten seconds before letting them go and holding them apart as naturally as possible. Notice the distance between them. How do your hands feel

now? What else do you notice in this moment? What's between your palms?

4   Interlock your fingers. Isn't that a remarkable geometrical institution? It's almost as if you've built your own cathedral with your hands. Which thumb is closer to you? Why, I wonder? Is that a bit of a thumby habit? How much pressure are you applying? Can you soften your cathedral just a little?

5   Do some finger flicks. Hold a hand out. Touch thumb and fore-finger first, make contact, add pressure and flick out. Repeat with each finger.

It might be useful in this moment to reflect on your expectations

So, how does this all sound? Fancy coming on a little journey with both me and your me? A mindful journal journey? We'll find out some things on the way and there will be plenty of opportunities for you to experiment with your own mindful journal practice. What do you say? You could use this moment to write about any expectations you have for yourself and your mindful journal practice.

Writing connects me up to the planets and the sun and the snow and my body

Whether I'm weary or upbeat, putting words to paper just works. Even if I'm stepping into my shadows – the darker sides to me, where difficulty resides – I'll feel different after the writing. There's science to back this up but I wouldn't even need science to tell me that, just as I don't need a peer-reviewed scientific study to tell me why hula-hooping is a lot of fun. Writing helps me renew my relationship with the world and my vows with courage and kindness. Ah, there goes courage – that great word – from the French *coeur*, for heart. Mindful journalling is none other than a work of heart.

Let's get started, but before we jump in . . .

I just wanted to let you know how I've written this book. Here are the three principles I've used throughout:

1 *You – dear reader–writer – already know how to journal mindfully, so just go and do it* Read this book to help you reflect on your own practice, by all means, but the wisdom is already in you. As with your wisdom teeth, you just need a bit of time and patience for your wisdom to come through, but it will come (and it can be painful). So write, right away. Go for it.

2 *If you have a body, you can write* Mindful journal practice is especially designed for people with bodies. Though we respect writer's block, we don't have much truck with it. Writer's block is about thinking. With mindful journalling, we don't think; we write, knowing we are writing. As Natalie Goldberg says, 'real writing comes from the whole body'. So we write from our body and all its glory. If we experience blockage still – even after moving from the mind to the body – we recognize it's a body blockage, so we simply move our position, or dance, or stand, or sit and wait, or do whatever the body wants us to do in this moment, allowing the blockage to be named (or at least acknowledged) and to break open. And if we still have writer's block – well, we just get up and do something else. Sometimes your body gets in the way, so you just have to go round it.

3 *Mindful journal writing is the same as all good writing* And good writing just means writing that's written with care and attention, writing that scares us (the word 'care' is hidden inside 'scare'; what scares us is what we care about). Good writing scares us but also enchants us. So the best guides for us as mindful journal writers – rather than me whispering ideas into your ears – are the mindful journals out there that exist in published form.

Take Henry David Thoreau's journal as a classic example: filled with forensic notation on his body, nature, philosophy, integrity, weather, animals, work, stillness, the habitat of habits and the passing of time. Thoreau's journal accompanied his daily walks, and charted his gloriously evolving selves and the passing seasons all at once – the seasons outside and the seasons inside.

There are loads of amazing mindful journals out there (and I include poems and other kinds of writing here) to inspire you, so check out:

- all the writings of Rumi and Hafiz;
- all the writings of Ralph Waldo Emerson and Henry David Thoreau;
- *Twelve Years a Slave* by Solomon Northup – an autobiography written with the courage and honesty we must find for mindful journalling;
- the diary of Anaïs Nin;
- the diary of Virginia Woolf;
- *The Book of Disquiet* by Fernando Pessoa;
- Elisabeth Bishop's poems and her gorgeously enormous *One Art: The selected letters*;
- the visual artist Keith Haring's journals – not at all mindful in ambition or scope, yet they're beautifully written and full of attentive awareness;
- the many volumes of journals by Trappist monk Thomas Merton (possibly my favourite kind of mindful journal; Thomas Merton's writing is a joy);
- *Walk Between Heaven and Earth* by Burghild Nina Holzer – I love her line: 'A journal can be anything! You hear me? A journal can be anything!'
- *Journal of a Solitude* by May Sarton;
- the poems of Mary Oliver – go and read 'Wild Geese' right away – and all her books, but especially her wonderful little *Long Life: Essays and other writing*;
- *A Time for New Dreams* by Ben Okri;
- *How the Light Gets In* by Pat Schneider – wonderful;
- *Modern Nature* – the journals of Derek Jarman;
- *Words Out of Silence: 60 days in solitude* by Bok (I urge you to read this extraordinary book);
- *Ongoingness* by Sarah Manguso.

These are just a few suggestions, and do find your own inspirations. At some level, you could just say that all great literature is mindful journal writing, because it's written by men and women who wrote as if their lives depended on it.

Write lying down

Lie on your back and allow yourself to do a gentle body scan from your big toes to the top of your head. Use a guided meditation CD or app to help you, if that's easier. During it, or afterwards, stay on your back and write in your mindful journal. So you're lying on your back, writing your mindful journal. Notice the sensations, the tug of gravity, the comfortableness, the strangeness of this. Vary it by lying on your front and writing in that position. What happens to your writing when you do this shift? What becomes easier? Notice where you go with words. As you are lying down, notice whether your words are telling the truth or, indeed, lying. Is it possible to tell your truth as you lie?

With this work, we are investigative journalists of the heart

I describe the mindful journal writer – you! – as an investigative journalist of the heart because it's so appropriate for what we're doing in this work. I prefer the metaphor 'investigative journalist' rather than, say, 'detective' because there's nothing to be resolved here, and everything to be revealed.

So like the investigative journalist, with mindful journalling:

- you're digging deep;
- the work takes time;
- it often starts with a tip-off;
- it can involve others and your relationship with them;
- it provides new knowledge;

- it operates at the level of depth, hiddenness and secrecy;
- and it relies on using multiple sources.

So go for it, my investigative journalist of the heart: go deep, go broad, go slow, go long. I wish you all the best as you begin to build, or rebuild, or simply bring awareness to, your mindful journal practice.

2

What is mindful journal practice?

There's nothing mysterious about this

Mindfulness is just about being in the present moment, with all that it holds, and accepting the present moment for what it is, no matter what it is.

And mindful journal practice, therefore, is that same process, but in written form. Mindful journalling can either refer to:

- writing about your *mindfulness practice*

or it can refer to

- writing about your *life* in a mindful way.

Either way, it doesn't matter: they're the same, because mindfulness isn't just a compartment of life, it is the whole of it.

Write as if your life depends on it

When I run writing workshops, I often give a writing prompt of some kind, before offering my writers a certain amount of time to write in. I like using eight-minute slots of writing time. I find it's enough to get something written down, and it's a short enough amount of time to have an inbuilt motivation system (biscuits are available). Plus, it's roughly the same amount of time it takes for sunlight to reach Planet

Earth, so that, in the writing, we've literally witnessed the passing of time and light itself. During the silence that accompanies the writing – generally there is silence, though there can be laughter, the odd gasp, a little wriggling – I sometimes allow myself some mindful people-watching and in this moment I notice two things happening: my writers are both doing and being.

Because my workshop is about bringing attention to the body in the act of writing, I have already given the writers prompts and invitations to use the hand crossing the page as another moment to experience life from the inside. So I know that I am watching people in the beautiful and paradoxical moment of practising both doing (the writing bit) and being (the mindfulness bit). In other words (a resonant phrase here), my writers are writing *through* their mindfulness practice. They're practising being by writing (ordinarily, a thing we call doing). But though they are not still, and though their writing looks a lot like doing, my writers are intentionally bringing their awareness to the page and their act of writing: they are *being* the writing. The invitation here is for you to do the same.

Breath and body are our best friends

In secular mindfulness, as it has been taught by pioneer teachers like Jon Kabat-Zinn, we learn to shift from the domain of doing to the domain of being. We learn to slow our bodies down and observe our minds and perceptions in a kind, calm and accepting way. We let thoughts come and go, we observe them; always, we gently guide ourselves back to the breath and the body.

We're not the White Rabbit in *Alice in Wonderland*, we don't rush down the rabbit hole after our thoughts. We just look at them, greet them, identify or label them (making them clearer, and therefore clearer not to be followed) and then let them go. In this moment, we return to our position – our sitting or standing meditation – and we continue to focus on the breath and our contact with the earth. Our breath and our bodies are our best friends in mindfulness (and especially mindful journalling).

Invite in the automatic pilot

How in touch with your body are you in this moment? Mindfulness is all about bringing awareness to all aspects of your lived experience, including – and especially – to your body, which can often be found in automatic pilot mode. I know mine certainly can be. Automatic pilot is essential, of course; we can't be aware of everything all the time. That would involve being in a continual state of meditation, which would itself become a kind of automatic pilot.

The key here is to befriend your automatic pilot, sit up front with him or her in the cockpit of your life, and invite kind curiosity to the bi-plane of your body–mind. With mindfulness, you can show your automatic pilot that there is so much more to this flying and living malarkey than just pressing some buttons and kicking back with a newspaper and a doughnut (apologies to any pilots reading this; I know you do a lot more than that).

To extend the metaphor, you can invite your pilot to take the handles once more, unclick the automatic pilot button and begin again to steer your life consciously and with mindfulness. Your pilot, now conscious pilot, sees new things, lives more deeply, experiences the airscape on his or her skin, observes thoughts for what they are – just thoughts. Rather than dwelling on past events or conjuring up future plans, your conscious pilot steers your life into open skies and existence through present, moment-to-moment attention, on purpose and without recourse to judgement.

With mindful journal practice we say hello to the inside and the outside of lived experience, and the bits in between

Mindful journalling is a kind of journalling that incorporates secular mindfulness – in the form that is taught in Mindfulness-Based Stress Reduction classes across the world – and teaches us how to bring awareness and attention to our writing: how to catch ourselves red-handed and red-hearted in the act of writing.

With mindful journal practice we move from doing-writing to being-writing by developing our own mindfulness practice alongside our journal practice. In this way, we can bring mindfulness to the writing act itself, so that the mindful journal writing itself becomes a kind of meditation practice. The act of writing, in this sense – the line of ink on the page – becomes a kind of breathing. With our mindfulness practice we can connect up with thousands of years of people sitting and breathing, just as in our mindful journal practice we can link up with thousands of years of people putting ink to page.

People have been mindful journalling for centuries

This work of stretching the imagination is not new by any stretch of the imagination. We've been mindful journalling for a long time:

- The Roman emperor Marcus Aurelius wrote his journals, published under the title *To Myself*, also *Meditations* (a potent word for us here), describing how to find and preserve equanimity at the heart of conflict.
- The Chinese philosopher Li Ao, heavily influenced by Buddhism, took a trip in 809 with his pregnant wife and journalled detailed descriptions of medieval southern China.
- The pillow books of Japanese court ladies, exemplified by Sei Shōnagon during the 990s (completed in 1002), are another fine example of early mindful journalling, particularly with their interest in the changing seasons and the 'pathos of things'.

- The earliest surviving Arabic diary, arranged in date order, is that of Ibn Banna in the eleventh century.
- The thirteenth-century writer Kamo no Chōmei wrote his *An Account of My Hut* in 1212, depicting the Buddhist concept of impermanence through the description of various disasters, such as earthquakes, famines and whirlwinds. The author moved further and further up into the mountains, eventually living in a 10-foot square hut located at Mt Hino. I love to think of us, as mindful journal writers, giving an account of our own huts – the huts of our first-person experience! So it's sweet, here, to think of your mindful journal as your very own *Account of Your Hut*. Why not write that title down in your journal and just carry on from there?
- Medieval mystics wrote about their bodily experiences of the presence of God, like Elisabeth of Schönau who journalled on wax tablets, later transcribed by her brother Egbert.
- The advent of the Renaissance and individualism saw the rise of the personal diary. One of the earliest preserved examples is the anonymous *Journal d'un bourgeois de Paris* that covers the lived experience of events between 1405 and 1449.
- The seventeenth-century Japanese poet Bashō wrote his travel diary, *Oku no Hosomichi* (literally: *Narrow Road to the Interior*), a collection of haibun (part diary, part haiku) that detailed in a concise way the changing states of both the writer and the world. I like the idea of your mindful journal as being a kind of 'narrow road to the interior'.

Though these might not be mindful journals as we're describing the practice in this book, these are certainly mindful journals in the sense that they were written by people

- living and writing as if their life depended on it;
- invested in notions of lived experience perceived from the big toes up;
- re-describing experience to connect to something bigger than themselves.

Literature can teach us so much about mindful journal practice

Here are some quotes from famous writers who kept diaries, alluding to the mindfulness of the practice:

Anaïs Nin:

> Over and over again I sail towards joy, which is never in the room with me, but always near me, across the way, like those rooms full of gayety one sees from the street, or the gayety in the street one sees from a window. Will I ever reach joy? It hides behind the turning merry-go-round of the travelling circus. As soon as I approach it, it is no longer joy. Joy is a foam, an illumination.

Anaïs Nin again:

> It was while writing a Diary that I discovered how to capture the living moments.

Virginia Woolf:

> I note however that this diary writing does not count as writing, since I have just re-read my year's diary and am much struck by the rapid haphazard gallop at which it swings along, sometimes indeed jerking almost intolerably over the cobbles. Still if it were not written rather faster than the fastest type-writing, if I stopped and took thought, it would never be written at all; and the advantage of the method is that it sweeps up accidentally several stray matters which I should exclude if I hesitated, but which are the diamonds of the dustheap.

André Gide:

> A diary is useful during conscious, intentional, and painful spiritual evolutions. Then you want to know where you stand . . . An intimate diary is interesting especially when it records the awakening of ideas; or the awakening of the senses at puberty; or else when you feel yourself to be dying.

Ralph Waldo Emerson:

> The good writer seems to be writing about himself, but has his eye always on that thread of the Universe which runs through himself and all things.

Oscar Wilde:

> I never travel without my diary. One should always have something sensational to read in the train.

Susan Sontag:

> Superficial to understand the journal as just a receptacle for one's private, secret thoughts – like a confidante who is deaf, dumb, and illiterate. In the journal I do not just express myself more openly than I could do to any person; I create myself. The journal is a vehicle for my sense of selfhood. It represents me as emotionally and spiritually independent. Therefore (alas) it does not simply record my actual, daily life but rather – in many cases – offers an alternative to it.

I love the singer-songwriter Sufjan Stevens. For me, his songs are the sung versions of mindful journal entries. I've been listening to lots of his albums while I've been writing this book. I recommend wholeheartedly finding music you can listen to either during your mindful journal writing or before and after. I feel at home with Sufjan's music in a way I feel at home in my mindfulness practice. Do any singers make you feel like that? For me, Sufjan embraces what Walt Whitman called both 'heart-singing and art-singing' and I wish both heart-writing and art-writing for us mindful journal writers.

We can all discover our own version of what Virginia Woolf meant by finding the 'diamonds in the dustheap'. For me, they're those sentences in your journal that melt your heart when you read them back; they surprise you, you thought someone else had written them (they hadn't, you did). I particularly warm to Susan Sontag's idea that we create ourselves in our journalling, that above confiding and confessing we nurture the new in ourselves, offer ourselves an alternative life to live. There are some lovely lines here, aren't there? I missed out about 80,000 other amazing quotations, including Pablo Picasso's 'Painting is just another way of keeping a diary' and William Wordsworth's 'Fill your paper with the breathings of your heart'; I like both of these because they remind me that breathing is beautiful and journalling gives me time and space to acknowledge that.

Do take a moment to reread them, take time with them and let them settle in your body. You could even copy one or two of your favourite quotes in your journal, like a commonplace book; a mindful journal is a great place to store great words and there are no rules, don't forget – just new ways to experiment with living a full and fantastic life.

There are seven foundational attitudes to mindful journal practice

Crucial to understanding mindfulness are the attitudes at the practice's foundation. Mindful journalling shares the same seven foundational attitudes of mindfulness itself, as conceived by Jon Kabat-Zinn. They are: non-judging, patience, beginner's mind, trust, non-striving, accepting, letting go. Like the stars and planets, they're interconnected, so working on one of the attitudes feeds all of the others. We'll come back to these, but here's an overview for now:

- *Journalling without judgement*: we have to be able to write sentences in our journal and not judge ourselves for them, just as we have to be able to allow thoughts to come without judging them in mindfulness.
- *Journalling with patience*: this practice won't come overnight. It takes time. Mindful journalling is like any art form in that way, including mindfulness itself.
- *Journalling with beginner's mind*: can we come to the blank page each time with fresh new eyes, without bringing any assumptions from past experience, or expectations about future experience? Can you constantly be a beginner-againer?
- *Journalling with trust*: it will get tough, and when the going gets tough, trust in the going.
- *Journalling without striving*: though it looks as though we're writing and striving to write, we're in fact meditating with pen and paper. With mindful journalling we're not trying to get anywhere or

be anything other than who we are in the magnificence of this moment.

- *Journalling with acceptance*: however we are in this moment, we journal it, and through that journalling we accept ourselves a little bit more. By writing things down, we accept them. The act of writing itself is the act of acceptance.
- *Journalling, then letting go*: by writing things down and closing our book, we accept our words and then let go of them. We can see the sentences – which relate to thoughts, feelings and bodily sensations – and in that seeing we let go. So we are free: this work is nothing if not radical.

Meditate on your pen

As a writer, your pen is a fantastic object to meditate on: so bring attention to your pen. Hold it in your palm. Feel its weight, the lightness, the density. Let some words describe the pen in your head or in your body. Note them without writing them down or following them. Hold your pen up to the light. Zoom in by bringing your pen nearer to one eye (the other might be shut). Hold it away from you. Notice your breathing in this moment. Breathing in, breathing out, noticing the gap between. Breathing in, breathing out, the gap between. Listen to your pen (hold it up to your ear). Feel the pen on your lips (careful for ink spillage or perhaps don't care about it!). Perhaps you can even balance the pen on your philtrum – the bit between your mouth and nose. Can you hold it there, no hands? Bring the pen back to the page. Start writing with it. Feel inside your hands, inside your fingers. What does it feel like from inside? Feel your hand move across the page. Do different words feel different to write? Write really quickly, slowly, scribble, scrawl, slow down, pause. Do a final full stop on the page, really slowly, as slowly as you can. Feel the full stop. Hear it. Meditate on the full stop. Then bring your hands together and bow towards the page, thanking it and your surroundings for holding you as you explored the interiority of your lived experience. As a mindful journal writer, you always have your mindfulness of pen as a resource to use. Writer's block? Pah, just use your pen – it's mightier than the sword.

There are plenty of reasons to keep a mindful journal

Just in case you need a reminder from time to time, here are some reasons to keep you on the straight and narrow to the interior:

- You can access your mindful journal any time, anywhere. Just like the breath, your mindful journal practice is always here. You can access it even when you can't access it. Don't have your journal to hand? Allow sentences to come to mind and body. Notice them. Have them appear inside you (where do they appear?). Hold them. Which ones will you recall later when you have your journal to hand? What is writing, after all? Is it the having-the-sentence-in-your-head-ready-to-be-written, or the actual act of writing it down? Are sentences fully formulated in our heads before they appear on the page or are they acts of improvisation in the moment? Can you breathe into that gap between thought and sentence a bit more? What happens when you hold a sentence a little longer in your head? Notice how you can write, even when you can't.

- Your mindful journal embodies the foundational attitudes of mindfulness. It accepts you for who you are, looks at you afresh with beginner's mind each time, holds your words with openness and trust, does not judge you as you write, and embodies equanimity at the heart of conflict. Your mindful journal, in this way, becomes your compassionate witness.

- Rereading your journal later on can help you grow by bringing awareness, over time, to patterns and habits of the mind, body, head and heart that you hadn't been able to observe at the time.

- Your mindful journal helps you notice thoughts as thoughts, sentences as sentences, words as words. In this sense, it helps you grow your mindful meditation practice as a whole by being another laboratory for examining how to live a full and fascinating life. Here's what I mean: during sitting meditation, you bring awareness to thoughts and notice yourself getting distracted by them, before gently bringing yourself back to the breath or body. In mindful journal practice, you get to see the thoughts written down in word form. It's easier not to be distracted by them, because you've already allowed and accepted them by writing them down.

- You can use your mindful journal to record your experience of your mindfulness meditations themselves, so that your journal becomes a place to store both specific details (whereabouts, dates, lengths of sessions) and bodily sensations (the fragility of the body, the longings of the heart, the wobbliness of your standing, and so on), not to mention any goals you have (intentions to attend silent retreats and so on).

- Writing about difficult and traumatic things has health benefits beyond just *feeling good* and *getting something off your chest*. Dr James Pennebaker has shown that writing about trauma for 15 minutes a day for four days can boost your immune system (more on this later). Richard Davidson, Jon Kabat-Zinn and others showed in 2003 that meditators who wrote about negative emotions experienced more activation in the left region of the brain – the area now associated with positive emotions – showing that they had learned to adapt well to unpleasant mind states; they also generated more antibodies after a flu vaccine than non-meditators. David Creswell's research showed that labelling emotions calms the brain: the amygdala, the part of the brain that sounds an alarm in times of danger, was less active in participants who looked at photos of people whose expressions were labelled 'angry', 'fearful' and so on.

- Your mindful journal practice can help bring awareness to your relationships with other people and, by reflecting on them or working with them creatively in written form, help bring mindfulness to opportunities for expansiveness within relationships. Writing the relationship into page can help soften the relationship in the 'real world', particularly with loving-kindness writing. Or, to paraphrase Susan Sontag, you can create the relationship anew through the journal writing.

- Your mindful journal can help you meditate on personal action and help you decide how to interact in society and politics for social justice ends. Your journal becomes, here, a meditation on power and subjugation, your objectification by the capitalist system (or whatever system you are forced under), if that's important to you. With mindfulness and agility, and equanimity, you can reduce suffering through awareness raising and investigative journalism of the heart and the state of things.

• Your mindful journal practice can help you get beyond yourself and into the more impersonal, numinous space of communion and connection with all beings, things and planets. Through mindful journal practice you find your place in what Mary Oliver calls 'the family of things'. You can connect with your wildness, your mystery, that uncertainty at your core. Your mindful journal is none other than a doorway through which you can step into the other side of the multiverse. Your mindful journal helps you make what Jon Kabat-Zinn calls the 'orthogonal shift'; it helps you move into, and be with, an earthly, shift-altering revolution of consciousness.

It's worth reflecting on why it is you want to keep a mindful journal. Did any of these reasons above resonate with you?

And use the close of this chapter, as you prepare for the next one, as another opportunity to feel grounded in your body (your feet firmly on the floor), to bring attention to your breath and eye contact with the page, and to feel present and in touch with your wholeness and the adventure you are embarking on. Are you ready to meet yourself? Come on, then.

3

Gathering – preparing to write your mindful journal

Turning on the journalling switch

Here's an exercise where I'll first ask you to imagine doing something and then I'll ask you to actually physically do it.

Imagine a simple, quiet room with a table and a chair in it, a window and some light. On the table rests your journal, and a pen beside it. Your journal is, in this moment, closed. There is no-one in the room. There are the sounds of birds outside. Holding this image in your heart, body and mind, you are about to walk into the room in the warmth of your imagination. You'll walk up to the table, pull out the chair slightly and sit down. You'll open your journal and take hold of your pen. Do this a few times. Stay with it. There's no need to rush.

Now that you have imagined this, have a go at doing it for real with intention and attention. So:

- place your journal on a table in a room;
- leave the room, then return to it;
- walk up to your journal with kindness;
- approach it as if you were approaching a little deer in the distance;
- find the mindfulness in the approach to your journal, whether it's for the first time or for the umpteenth time.

What did you notice? Use this brief moment to jot down some thoughts relating to this exercise, noting any differences between the act of imagination and the physical act of actually doing it. How are you approaching your journal today? Might it have something to do with how you're approaching your life today?

Turning on the journalling switch means carving out time and space, intentionally

I call it the journalling switch because I'm too impressed by what Anat Baniel calls 'the learning switch' to find my own way of saying it. Joyfully, a journalling switch and a learning switch are much the same. Anat Baniel trained in Feldenkrais – a technique that explores awareness through movement – and she now teaches her own NeuroMovement method, which is all about helping people live with strength, flexibility and vitality: given strength, flexibility and vitality are going to be incredibly useful for us mindful journal writers – after all, mindful journalling involves a lot of awareness through movement – I've used some of her ideas in this book. I wholeheartedly recommend her book, *Move into Life*, to you.

Back to the learning switch

I think it's crucial for us to use this practice of mindful journalling as a way of dedicating ourselves to our own lifelong learning pathway. Mindful journal practice is mindfulness-inspired self-study. At some level, our mindful journal is a record of what we've learned, but it is also – through the awareness brought to the writing itself – an experience of learning in its own right; it is an experience of the learning itself unfolding. And, perhaps even more importantly, it is a record of our *intentions* to record the patterns of our attention from moment to moment. You could say, the lifelong learning is in this very capturing of moment-to-moment experience as it unfolds on the page.

When you approach mindful journalling, you approach mindful learning

Baniel uses the vitality of a child as her inspiration for what's really behind the learning switch. Child-like vitality is something we can each reach again by turning on the learning and the journalling switch. Here's the analogy:

- It's easy to notice how a child plays in the world, how she engages with things with fresh new eyes, asking questions we might never have thought of ourselves because we were too busy lugging the shopping bags from the boot of the car. The vital child contrasts with the unmindful adult, who – in this story anyway – has forgotten how wonderful the sky looks at dusk, has got into a rut, has assumed things were the way they were (and possibly always will be), has finally begun to believe the propaganda of his habitual responses.

Baniel uses the story of the explorer Ferdinand Magellan to make her point about learning, which I'm suggesting is relevant to us as we gather ourselves together for mindful journalling:

- When Magellan sailed across the Pacific Ocean (he called it the 'peaceful sea'), he completed the first circumnavigation of the earth.
- When he and his crew landed on the Pacific islands, the 'natives' (as he would have called them) asked them how they had got there.
- So just imagine it for a second. The large ships in which the crew had arrived were right behind them on the horizon and the 'natives' were still wondering how they got there; the explorers surely would have just pointed at the ships and said to the 'natives', 'But can't you see?'
- Well, no, the point is – the 'natives' couldn't see the ships: they were invisible to the indigenous people. They didn't have the same brain wirings as the Europeans to be able to identify 'ship-ness'. They weren't *ready* to see the ships. Imagine likewise what the

explorers couldn't see, too, what I can't see, what you can't see right now. That could be today's journal entry: 'Things I cannot see today'.

Mind the pun, but: do you see? In other words, when we have a kind relationship with our own faculty for learning and seeing new things, we become more transparent; our whole body becomes fuller and we are more able to engage with the world, more able to see both what we can see and what we can't. So with mindful journalling we play the role of both explorer and 'native'. We switch on our learning and journalling switch – saying yes to possibility – and practise mindful attention towards what is always already here.

What are your intentions with keeping your mindful journal?

Why not spend a page or so writing them down? You might like to answer some of the following questions, or just list 'Ten things I want to achieve with my mindful journal':

- Who am I writing this for?
- What do I want to happen after six months of keeping my mindful journal?
- What kinds of thing will I record? Experiences from my day? Sensory perceptions from key moments in my day? Plans for the coming week? Things I'm grateful about? Things on my mind?
- How will I regard my shadow when it crosses my journal? Will I go there or will I steer clear?
- What kind of book am I writing here?
- Will I include dreams from the night before as well as dreams for the future?
- Who might read my mindful journal?
- How might keeping a mindful journal help me be in the present moment?
- What do I long for?

Mindful journalling helps you shift from *previous* ways of attending to *precious* ways of attending

To be able to turn on the journalling and learning switches, we simply have to be open to seeing giant ships on our own horizon. We embrace an attitude of learning and being with both the knowing and the not knowing. It's all down to our brilliant brains. They're geared to do things efficiently, but all too often

- 'efficiently' becomes 'doing things repeatedly',
- which is all well and good until 'doing things repeatedly' becomes 'doing things repeatedly *for their own sake*'.

When there is a new activity – like kite-flying, for example – our brains quickly create a huge number of new synapses. 'We become vibrant,' says Baniel, just like the child, astonished by her learning. But over time, our brain realizes we don't need certain synapses, so it gets rid of them and chooses the most efficient path. This is called pruning.

It's necessary, of course, but pruning has its own problems. With repeated experiences of the same thing, the plastic brain tends to want to reject any neurons that might upset the apple cart and alter the pattern of synapses. In other words, the brain – once it has learnt the new skills – has an inbuilt tendency to resist any new learning related to it; it just wants to do that one thing, and do it very well. The brain that had once whooped with excitement at the new activity now wants to get so good at that new activity that it gets stuck in a groove. The brain would prefer the groove to survive above all else.

This is where we come in – the person with the brain

More important than grooves for their own sake – continually grooving on and on – is a healthy balance of:

- pleasure and
- mastery promoted by

- an attitude of lifelong learning that is achieved through
- activity and curiosity paired with
- gentle pausing, slowing down and noticing our breathing.

So when we say hello to our ability to learn new things – potentially at any stage across the life course thanks to the plasticity of our brains – we're sending out the signal to our brain and body that we're still here, that we're more than just the safety of repeated, groove-based activity.

It's the same with our mindful journal practice

It's crucial not to get in a rut with this work; or rather, this work is essentially about not getting in a rut. Each time we approach our mindful journal, it's important to inhabit that foundational attitude of beginner-againer's mind – the one you practised at the beginning of this chapter. By writing yourself into learning, by opening your palms and heart and falling for the lifelong mystery of yourself, you begin to transform yourself each time you step into the wild.

Each time you come to your journal, prepare to write with gentleness; slow down, pause, become a conscious inhabitant of your body, feel yourself in your chair, sitting slap-bang in the middle of your life, knowing you are doing so. This is, after all, writing, knowing the writing, *being* the writing that knows.

Turning on the journalling and learning switches involves this conscious act of slowing down

So here we are in Gathering mode. Before you even write anything in your journal today, can you slow down? Can you do the little ritual we did right at the start of this chapter and attend to yourself in the act of the approach? Accompany yourself to your journal, the way a new guest might be accompanied to his or her room at a hotel. Sit on the bed and test your new room first, before jumping right in.

Non-judging is the thing (aka kindness)

Mindfulness involves kindly stepping back from the chatter of thoughts and judgements in your head and allowing yourself to just be with them as you fall fully into your body. We sit on the banks and watch our thoughts pass us by in a happening as beautiful and natural as a river. And of course, if we start judging our thoughts, which is as natural as a river, rather than beating ourselves up for that, we just observe the judging with kindness, and bring our attention gladly back to the interested noticing mode (as opposed to the involved swept-up one). The key with mindfulness is awareness, so that even if we 'break the rules' of mindfulness, we can still use our flouting as an opportunity to explore lived experience from all angles.

Mindful journalling requires non-judging, especially in the act of writing down words, not letting the inner critic throw them in the bin before you've even had a chance to read them back to yourself. The investigative journalist of the heart does not throw balls of scrunched-up paper in the bin. If anything, he sends out party invitations.

Mindful journalling involves practising patience

We don't have to rush with this work of mindfulness and mindful journal practice. Patience is the wisdom that kindness and slowing down, and not trying to push the river or get to the next moment, reveal so much more. There is so much going on even in one single moment – tensions in the body, pressure through contact with the floor, the background hum of thinking and judging, the emerging of a felt sense of here and now – that even if we can slow down and be patient for just one of those moments, we're doing some really good work here.

Mindful journal practice requires patience on the page. Sometimes words don't come to us so quickly or carefully, and we think we're writing rubbish. If we can be patient with our writing selves, if we can wait just that little bit longer before writing the next word, perhaps we can expand our possibilities for spaciousness and word-fulness. Patience and non-judging are close friends for the mindful journal writer, both enabling each other to take hot air balloons into the sky of your heartfelt imagination.

With this work, you embrace beginner-againer's mind

A central tenet of mindfulness and mindful journalling is beginner's mind (it's very much related to our journalling and learning switches). Here, as we gather ourselves for mindful journal practice, we embrace beginner's mind: aka *looking afresh at the world each time*. How often do we see the same things in our daily lives, attend the same rituals (travelling to work, meeting the same people and so on)? We could easily assume we *know* these people, the same things we see. But how much do we really know these familiar things? What's different and new inside same old, same old?

With mindfulness practice, we start again (or even start to start again); we bring freshness and newness to our experience and our experience of experience:

- However you find yourself in this moment, reading this page (which looks so similar, doesn't it, to all those other pages), can you bring beginner-againer's mind to your inner experience?

- When you write your mindful journal, can you experience afresh the feel of pen landing on paper, the emergence of words across the page, the soft transcription of thought into sentence?

- Books often have a preface, and I find that a useful word in this context. The preface is where we begin to begin. What do you need to do before you face up to your writing today?

Feel the gravitational pull on you as you begin to write; feel your poise

Gathering mode involves an awareness of gravity. Once you are sitting in your chair, ready to write in your journal, it is worth noticing – even very briefly – gravity's graceful pull on you towards the centre of the earth. There is no way we can even conceive of experience as we know it without gravity. Even our experience of a lack of gravity – for most of us through watching astronauts on TV – is premised on a fundamental familiarity with being constantly pulled down.

Gravity can teach us about attraction and consistency

And it has much to say about providing security and opening up physical possibilities. With gravity, we know where we are, we can find ourselves in physical and more heartfelt ways. We learn about our heaviness, sinking feelings, but also our unbearable lightness. Often we drop something and it smashes or breaks; do we blame or thank gravity in these moments? Gravity is as defining of experience as it is revealing. We can but dance in it. In gravity, we discover our poise.

Without really knowing it, we're all gravity experts. Even just walking forwards involves a complex interrelationship within and between our entire body and the universe. Gravity is what Moshe Feldenkrais would count as 'the elusive obvious'. It is there but it is not there. Bringing our attention to it, just before we write our mindful journal entries, is another radical act of love. We can write about gravity in our mindful journal, or just pay attention to it as we write. Either way, gravity pours into our mindful journal practice. It is never far away, much like light and breathing, inking and linking. So in this moment, take a photograph of your relationship with gravity and stick it into your mindfulness journal.

With this work, you are enquiring into what it is possible and pleasurable, permissible and plausible

Before you begin writing your mindful journal in any particular day you might find it useful to let these questions settle inside you:

- What is it possible for me to write about today? What is impossible for me to write about today?
- What is pleasant for me to write about today? What is unpleasant for me to write about today?
- What is permissible for me to write about today? What is impermissible for me to write about today?
- What is plausible for me to write about today? What is implausible for me to write about today?

What is the difference between all these words? Some might seem similar, though there are subtleties involved in each. That which is possible to write about might well be pleasurable to write about. Just because I may write about it, is it within my character to? Is what is possible to write about plausible for me to write about? What does plausible even mean here? Is it pleasurable to write about something no-one would expect you to write about? Are there some things that I wouldn't expect myself to write, that other people wouldn't expect me to write, but that I could still write?

Find your own take on these P-words. They're underneath all writing (and reading, of course); they underpin the whole of literature. I wonder if great writing might occur when writers write what's impossible, unpleasant, impermissible and implausible for them to write. I wonder if sticking with the known, the possible, the pleasurable, the permissible is fine too. What balance can we strike? You could even write those questions in your journal today and answer them. List things for each question. This will create a fantastic resource for future writing.

As you gather yourself to write, reflect on the possibility of encountering difficulty in this work

The poet Mary Oliver, very much a gentle guide for me with this wonderful mindful journal work, writes that darkness – what we might call our shadow, or just *things we find difficult in this moment* – is 'a gift'. I think it is incredible to think of our darkness in this way – as a beautifully wrapped present to be unfolded, understood, loved even – and the invitation to you, likewise, is to consider your own darkness a gift, however difficult – especially however difficult. After all, whenever you walk in the sun, you gain a shadow. So here, as we gather ourselves, we reflect on difficulty.

You always have a choice with mindful journal practice about whether or not you want to write about the difficulty

If you do, the research shows that writing about difficult things has therapeutic benefits, including increased ability to accept your situation and an improved immune system. If you don't want to, bringing kind mindful awareness to your edge today, and your sense that you cannot cross it, is certainly good enough.

Go slowly, with kindness, and you can't go wrong. This is why meditation practice is so important alongside your mindful journal practice. You'll find that your meditation and mindful journalling practice helps you distinguish more easily the difference between thoughts, emotions and bodily sensations, which in turn helps you go up slowly to conclusions, rather than rush to them, if you find you reach any conclusions at all.

Being with difficulty is part of what that great thinker, writer and Quaker Parker J. Palmer calls 'living the questions', using Rilke's line. When you live the questions, you go up close to difficulty and find the 'hidden wholeness' at the heart of yourself. You find you can live 'divided no more' and you 'let your life speak'. I love Parker Palmer's work, and – like the work of Anat Baniel and Jon Kabat-Zinn which I've used to help listen into speech some of this stuff around mindful journal practice – I couldn't recommend it enough to you. Details of all the books I've used are at the back.

If it gets too difficult, stop. Journal with ease

So as we gather ourselves, preparing to mindfully journal, we can reflect on our relationship with difficulty:

- If it's just too difficult, we stop. We don't continue writing. We ask ourselves, 'What do I need in this moment?' And we step away and nourish ourselves in whatever way we need that's safe and helpful.
- Or, if you can do some writing but not much, just write down the labels for your thoughts (rather than the contents), like this: 'Difficult thought, sad memory, sad memory, nice feeling . . .'
- Or write about what it is like having a shadow, but without describing the contents of the difficulty.
- Can you come up with a useful metaphor for your darker material?
- What might happen if you did write even just a bit of it down? What's the first line of the novel of your sadness? Could you edge a little closer into your shadow by writing just a sentence about the difficulty? And tomorrow, perhaps another sentence? You'll know what to do.

Trust in your body and your mindful journal practice and you'll be right as rain.

With wild journalling, we shift from antagonist to agonist

With mindful journal practice, we accept ourselves for whatever we are, for whatever we bring to the journal. Rather than wrestling with ourselves, we sit next to ourselves and listen to something breathing, something emerging, something writing. In this sense, we shift from being antagonistic with ourselves to being *agonistic* with ourselves.

Agonism is great. It's a bit like the word 'agony', which doesn't have great connotations for most people. When we become agonists, we have a deep respect and concern for ourselves and other people. The agon was the Ancient Greek athletic contest, where struggle and conflict were matched by generosity and admiration. I can see why in everyday speech we refer to agony as great physical anguish, but we seem to have stripped out the great bits of the struggle for victory too. Perhaps by mindful journalling we can go up close to all aspects of our lives and investigate them for what they are.

Mindful journal practice is built on trust

Along the way, along the path of mindfulness meditation and your mindful journal practice, it is highly likely that you will think you've come a cropper. I just wrote that without thinking it, and I'm tickled pink with that classic British idiom – 'to come a cropper'. Originally a phrase to describe falling off your horse, 'to come a cropper' means you've failed in some way. The good news with mindfulness and mindful journal practice is that it's very difficult, if not impossible, to come a cropper. Non-judging comes in here, of course – to think you've failed is to judge yourself – and trust becomes your newest ally, riding in on its own mindful horse.

Trusting yourself and your body is a lifelong practice and one essential to your mindful journal project. As you write, particularly if you're practising free writing (more on this later), use trust to help you be with the difficulty of feeling as if you've come a cropper. Not sure what to write? Trust yourself, the words will come (and if they don't, great!). Trust is the antidote to the propaganda of writer's block. Trust will happen as you build your practice, trust me. Writing trustfully and truthfully, without writing yourself off, is at the heart of mindful journalling.

There is nothing to strive for: you are already there

When we write our mindful journals, we don't need to be anywhere else nor do we need the writing to get us anywhere else. We're exactly where we should be. We're not writing to solve something, or to achieve anything, or to get published, or to finish a story or a poem. If kissing is what psychoanalyst Adam Phillips calls 'aim-inhibited eating', then mindful journalling is aim-inhibited writing. Yes, we might be creating a grand resource of words and sentences and turns of phrase that we can use in other things later (be they shopping lists, poems, eulogies . . .) but our mindful journal is – thankfully and beautifully – a place with no beginnings, no middles and no ends. We write *in media res* – in the middle of things, in the middle of our life. We might even say we write in the middle of the middle of things. And so, talking of writing, let's move on. We've gathered enough; now's the time to get jotting.

4

Jotting – writing your mindful journal entries

Just start writing

See what happens. What's the worst (and best) that can happen? Notice what you find yourself writing about: something that happened in the past, something that's happening now, something that might happen in the future, always grounded in the present moment through your breath and body, your hand pushing across the page. And so bear in body those foundational mindfulness attitudes:

- bring beginner-againer's mind to the blank page;
- be patient as your words come out;
- don't try to judge them in any way;
- trust the process and your practice;
- try not to reach anywhere (you're here, which is enough);
- accept yourself, accept your words, accept what interests you in this moment, let it be, let it be;
- and then let it go, let it go, let go of your pen, let go of this moment of writing.

See what happens. What's the worst and best that can happen?

Wait – this is all well and good, but what if I've got writer's block?

So it's good – at the start of Jotting mode, the second main feature of mindful journal practice – to reflect on writer's block, that classic stifling symptom that apparently affects writers everywhere. I'll use an example from real life to explain my theory that, with mindful journal practice at least, there is no such thing as writer's block.

There is no such thing as writer's block, just writer's body

I was recently in a writing workshop for people who have a yoga practice. Halfway between writing about an animal we've loved and standing up in mountain pose or tadasana (I always hear it as Ta-Da!-sana), I found myself saying to the group: 'Remember, there is no such thing as writer's block, just writer's body.'

I reckon I'm on to something

I guess my point is: this 'wild, silly and wonderful writing practice' (as Natalie Goldberg calls it) is always available to us, even when we don't think it is – and especially when we don't think at all.

We might say that the body is always here in the same way Freudians might say there is always the unconscious. So use it! Got writer's block? Head straight to your body! Start relocating today!

When it comes to embodied writing, impossibility is impossible

In this moment, even if there is nothing else, there is the opportunity to focus on the felt sense of my hands writing along the page, the lived experience of sitting in this chair, the feel of the air on skin. Let's focus on the hand. Call it beginner's hand: we can write about how it feels to make marks on paper, the hand travelling the page, how to experience difficulty making meaning. There is no block, if you have a body. Writing, like meditation, is an opportunity to come up close to this moment.

There is no such thing as writer's block, just the next sentence

Sentences to the writer are like moments to the mindfulness practitioner. They are things we can bring awareness to. From moment to moment, sentence to sentence.

The Wikipedia page for Writer's Block (yes, there is one) says that writer's block may result from a shift in the writer's brain from the cerebral cortex (consciousness, thought, language) to the limbic system (emotion, behaviour, memory), without the writer realizing it.

This makes me laugh. It's as if the tall, whimsical dandy of the cerebral cortex gets uppity and throws the writer's pen into the swamp of the deeply engrained fight-or-flight limbic system! Which is another way of saying, 'I can't write because I've hidden my pen from myself.'

Got writer's block? Give yourself lines

So if you do come up against difficulties that you suppose are writer's block – that seem to hinder the letting come of the writing – bring awareness to the blockage and invite it in. Say 'Welcome' to your block – whether it's a thinking writer's block or a limbic body block – and write again and again in your journal: 'Welcome, blockage' or 'Welcome, bit of me that can't write in this moment' or just simply 'Welcome'. Do this again and again and again. It's a bit like lines – that awful punishment at school that was given in 'detention'. So if you get writer's block, give yourself a gorgeous, gentle detention: write again and again and again a welcoming sentence. In your little detention, bring attention to the curious feel of the hand crossing the page; notice your breathing, your posture, your relationship of eye to paper. It could well be that you effortlessly shift from writing your welcome lines to continuing your mindful journal entry. But if detention doesn't help, mindfully move your body or go and do something completely different instead. It could well be the wisdom of your body knowing in advance of you that right now is not a time to write. 'Later, later,' your body whispers to you, 'you will write again later.'

The limbic system is a great place to write!

And anyway, writers don't write with their cerebral cortex just as much as they don't write with their limbic systems. They write with their hands, with their breath, their bodies, their movement, their hidden wholeness.

With our mindful journal practice we become experts of starting again

Each blank page is an invitation to turn up. There is no such thing as writer's block here because we can always describe simply and kindly – without judgement and with patience – the felt sensations of writer's block, and that – it is highly likely – will set us off into a new direction. The writer's block becomes our best friend if we welcome it into us as a friendly part of us. In describing its outline – the silhouette of our inarticulacy – we move through it into wordfulness. As my mindfulness teacher Lorraine says, you can't be anxious if you're curious.

So when you start writing, you are entering a new space or time, you are beginning again (and not necessarily beginning at the beginning). You are literally writing mindful journal *entries* – so this is entry-level work, no matter how expert you are. And entries are entrances, they're thresholds, they're things to enter, to penetrate. Who and what you are entering is up to you, but it is worth knowing that this work is about getting to the heart of something. With mindful journal practice you have to admit that you will get to the heart of the matter, and you will get closer to the heart of the matter, and you (or we might say all of you) matter. In other words, it will change you.

And if you've still got writer's block?

Always blame your tools. Pretend your pen's run out and go and run out with it. Do something else. It's just silly mindful journal writing.

The practical mindful journal writing exercises

The rest of this chapter consists of practical mindful journal writing exercises. So although the invitation is just to write, however writing comes, it can be useful, sometimes, to be guided. Here's a little list of the exercises you will find in this chapter to help you with your mindful journal entries (it also acts as a checklist you can tick as you try each practice). And there are 31 writing exercises in total, one for each day of the month:

1 Write in mindfulness meditation
2 Write using Naikan practice
3 Write with gratitude
4 Write with your whole body
5 Write with plain language
6 Write using free writing
7 Write with ununderstanding
8 Write using memory
9 Write using improvisation
10 Write using dialogue
11 Write a list of nouns
12 Write letters to your selves
13 Write with subtlety
14 Write about the quality of light
15 Write using the steppingstones method
16 Write borrowing opening lines from great poets
17 Write with Focusing
18 Write your famous last words
19 Write about objects in front of you
20 Write out your loving kindness meditation

21 Write a story about your breath
22 Write your virtues or values
23 Write using bibliomancy
24 Write in front of a mirror
25 Write using Sei Shōnagon's lists
26 Write using double-entry journalling
27 Write what you hear
28 Write sentences that begin with 'Hello'
29 Write about three different kinds of experience
30 Write with your eyes shut
31 Write without writing.

So give these exercises a try, not worrying too much, and being super-generous to yourself. If you want to time yourself, try writing in eight-minute slots; as we noticed before, it's roughly the same amount of time it takes for sunlight to reach earth, so it feels like a beautiful, useful amount of time. But equally, don't worry about timing yourself; you could spend a day doing lots of these exercises. And don't forget some of the things we talked about earlier:

- Vary your approach to elicit different kinds of writing; so tweak the exercise or vary how you're sitting or standing.
- Go subtler to find the hidden words under your words; slow down; pause; give yourself time to find the details; don't forget you're investigating yourself.
- After each exercise, ask yourself: what have I learned about myself today? What do I find here? What is here? What might be underneath these words?
- If something's too difficult, pause the writing, or change what you're writing about, or do some physical movement or meditation to vary your position.
- Check your awareness; at any time you can always bring your awareness back to your breath or to your hand moving across the page or your gravitational pull. Are you still there, writing and knowing you are writing?

1 Write in mindfulness meditation

With mindfulness, there are four main meditations, also known as dignities. These are:

- Sitting meditation
- Standing meditation
- Lying down meditation (also the body scan)
- Walking meditation.

The invitation here is to approach your meditation as ever you normally would – gently, with kind attention to yourself and your surroundings, focusing on the breath and bringing attention back to the breath whenever the mind wanders – but with one difference: you keep your journal next to you. In this way, at any time you can write down in your journal notes that arise from your practice. You might find it a useful way of bringing your attention back from thoughts to the breath – by writing them down first! You can either write during the meditation or just before or after it: it's up to you, and each way will bring up different kinds of writing.

2 Write using Naikan practice

Bring a bit of Japanese Naikan practice into your mindful journal. Naikan – literally meaning 'introspection' or 'looking in' – is a structured method of self-reflection developed by businessman and devoted Jodo Shinshu Buddhist Yoshimoto Ishin. Naikan can help you understand yourself and your relationships better and I reckon it can also be a great tool for your mindful journal practice. Here's how to use it.

Think about someone. Naikan traditionally begins with your mother but you can think about anyone – a friend, a colleague, a relative. Now that person's in your mind's eye, write down each of these questions in your journal, and then answer them:

1 What have I received from this person?
2 What have I given to this person?
3 What troubles and difficulties have I caused to this person?

You might think I've missed out the question: 'What troubles and difficulties has this person caused me?' But in fact the method is genius because it pre-supposes you know those things already.

Naikan is really special. It suggests that we do lovely things for those who cause us difficulty, which is counter-intuitive, of course (though I wonder why). Reflection and contemplation is the key, and your mindful journal is a great place for you to hold various Naikan-style reflections on people you are in relationship with.

3 Write with gratitude

Write down three things you're really grateful about from today. Give details, if you can. Be specific. If you're grateful to the person who held open the door for you while you had your arms full, who was it, what was it he or she said, what was the overall colour of the scene, what happened next, what did the person smell like, how did your heart feel?

Got more than three? Write as many as you can. Isn't there so much to be grateful for? Can you be grateful for difficult things? Can you acknowledge difficulty here and find the thing to be grateful for within the difficulty? Is there always something to be learned, even (perhaps especially) in the shadowy parts of our day? What can't you be grateful for today? List those things too. And what would you like to be grateful for tomorrow? List those things too.

4 Write with your whole body

When you write your mindful journal, what is doing the writing? Your hand? Well, a hand can't write without thoughts to turn into sentences. So you must be using your mind, or at least certainly your brain, as well. But to get your brain going you need oxygen from your lungs and blood from your heart. And you need a skeleton to rise out of the earth, and feet and buttocks to give you support, and fat and muscles and . . . You get the idea. It's the whole of you that is doing the writing.

When you write, reflect on this fact that it is the whole of you, and the wholeness of you – what Parker J. Palmer calls the 'hidden wholeness' of you – that writes. So write from the point of view of every part of you. This task will take a lifetime. Start today: write with your big toes. What are they saying? Then move up your whole body. Write an entry on what your knees are telling you, your crotch, your upper back, your neck, your eyebrows . . . Here's how you could approach each body part with enquiry:

- Eyes: what do they see? What do you see when you look at them in the mirror? How do eyes feel in this moment? What happens to your breath when they look at different things? What can you see in your life in this moment?

- Knees: these hinges are crucial for sitting down and standing up and walking. Practise each and notice the quality of knee. Knees might be about your needs. What do you need in this moment?

- Small of your back: that lovely unexplored area around your lower back can be curved and soft. You can't really see it without a mirror, but perhaps you can use your mindfulness powers to experience your small in other ways. How is small today? How small do you feel in this moment? How could you feel larger?

- Other questions: What do your cells want to write in this moment? What do the nuclei in your cells want to journal in this moment? Can you experience your diaphragm? What do your fascia – the connective tissue fibres beneath your skin that separate muscles and organs – have to say? What kind of support does your skeleton need in this moment? What words could match the experience of skeleton?

5 Write with plain language

Sometimes, you will just want to write your mindful journal entry as if you are taking a photograph. In this sense, you want the page to hold a truthful version of the day's events (as truthful as any good camera, I mean) and nothing more. To do this, you need to practise the art of using plain language. It's a lovely thing to do and really goes to the heart of mindful journalling.

You might like to use this simple language approach when writing about your meditation practice, for example, or a wonderful meeting with a friend (or even a difficult one). I love to meditate on my Fortescue drum in the middle of my front room, opposite the window, out of which I can see the Baptist Chapel and the tops of some buildings. If I want my journal to reflect the plainness of my experience, I just say it as it is: I journal about the light coming through the window and the shadows it makes on the wall. I write about the orange leaves falling outside the window (specific details like this, that don't stray into metaphor too much, are really helpful). I use language that is very spare, very simple and very evocative. I explore the feelings below my skin using simple language, as if I'm photographing myself from every angle. There are few metaphors, if any. There might be similes, but they're very simple ('The sky was blue, like at the sea'). I try and use plain language to describe things as they are.

I love this work, because we can find the simple and the sacred in the secular and the everyday, and plain language is just as good as ornamental (if not better). Try this now. Write about something from your day using the plainest language possible. It's like putting a vase of flowers on the table in your heart, walking away and then turning around to have a good look.

6 Write using free writing

Free writing is the best proof that there is no such thing as writer's block, or if there is at least it's your best friend. You write in blocks of time (I generally use eight minutes) without lifting your hand off the page. You can write about anything (rule one) but you can't not write (rule two). If you need help with the first line, borrow one from a book (randomly plucked), or use this: 'I love this moment because . . .' or 'This moment is . . .' If you run out of things to say, just write, 'I don't know what to write right now, I don't know what to write right now, I don't know . . .' until you're off again.

Free writing is a great way to bring attention to your hands and eyes and their contact apart and together, and to your thoughts and your words in relationship. When time's up, read back your words, underline your favourites or lines that intrigue you about yourself, then start again, using one of those lines as your next first line. Free writing is a great way of writing your mindful journal or building a resource of words for the future, and it's a tool you've always got to hand.

7 Write through your unundertanding

The wonderful writer Grace Paley describes writers as needing to write because, while they think they're specialists on life, they don't understand a thing about life; so they write to understand it, but it never becomes clear – hence the endlessness and the bottomlessness of the need to write. I think you'll empathize with that as much as I do. So, as Paley says, the writer 'takes his ununderstanding . . . and never gets over it'.

So why not take your ununderstanding and never get over it – mindfully? Write a list of all the things you don't understand. Each sentence can start something like 'I don't understand . . .' Bring attention to your breath and your heart as you do so. List all that you do not get. Go for it. A whole world of not knowing is your oyster!

8 Write using memory

Does a day go by when we don't have a visit from a memory? When they come, use them as ways into mindful journal writing. Memories can be difficult, of course. They can be vague and blurry, so difficult to remember or recall exactly. They can be about difficult times in our lives, and so perhaps we only allow ourselves to go into the details when we feel strong or safe. Joe Brainard's book *I Remember* is a fantastic inspiration here. The book is made up of sentences where each line begins 'I remember . . .' followed by the thing he remembers. If a memory doesn't come naturally, I recommend this no-brainer Joe Brainard approach.

Write 20 lines where each line begins 'I remember . . .' Try to remember different kinds of things, from different epochs in your life. Write 100 if you can. You'll find you've got many more memories than you thought you had. As ever, check in with your body, feel the breath accompanying each memory, the flow and the pace of breathing and remembering. If a memory comes naturally, hold it in meditation, observe it with kind distance, let it be – don't necessarily follow it, just let it settle – and then write from that new place of seeing and being with memory.

9 Write using improvisation

I've been going to some improvisation workshops and the most important thing you learn is the 'Yes, and . . .' technique. It's a wonderful one and has helped me in lots of aspects of my life. If someone offers you something, you 'Yes, and . . .' it – so for example, if someone says, 'Here, I've got you a present' (they've got nothing in their hands, we're improvising), you say, 'Oh wonderful, I always wanted an alarm clock' (you both now pretend you have an alarm clock in your hands), and they then say, 'Yes, it's a lovely big red alarm clock, isn't it?' and you say, 'Yes it is. It's funny, but I never thought I'd need a big red alarm clock that I could also scrunch up into my pocket' (scrunching it up and putting it in your pocket), to which they then say, 'Yes, it's so good, it vibrates your leg when the alarm goes off' (audience laughs) and you then shake your leg (more laughter) – and so on. You get the idea.

In improv, we never say never, just as in mindful journal practice: we just say yes, and then build on it. I recommend this as a writing strategy for your mindful journal (and, while we're at it, life). Here's how you could use 'Yes, and . . .' in your journal:

- Start by writing a sentence that describes something truthful and honest about your day. For example, 'Today I sat by the window, drinking ginger tea.'

- Then, write the next sentence by starting it with 'Yes, and . . .' and finish the sentence with something else – it can be truthful but it can also be fabricated or entirely imaginary, just so long as it builds on the previous sentence. So, for example, you might then write, 'Yes, and then I thought about that time we ran down to the beach with Nate the dog.'

- And then you start the next line with (you guessed it) 'Yes, and . . .' and build up the story, doing so again and again so that each line is a continuation and a building on from the last.

- You'll end somewhere completely different from where you started. You'll surprise yourself, I guarantee.

How else can you bring an attitude of 'Yes, and . . .' into your life and journal writing? Have a go at some of these (write them in your journal and improvise your answers):

- Is it perhaps equally mindful to 'Actually, no . . .' something?
- What is your relationship with yeses and noes in this moment?
- Who last said yes to you and who last said no?
- Where does yes come for you in your body? Practise nodding your head a few times. Slow it down, speed it up. Vary your nods and then use your felt experience to write in your journal.

- Where does no appear? What's the relationship between your noes and your nose?
- Write journal entries where you list all the things you say yes to and all the things you say no to.

10 Write using dialogue

Writing dialogue in your mindful journal is a lovely way to record your experience mindfully. You could recall a conversation from your day, for example, or make up a conversation. You could be an investigative journalist and interview your body parts, part by part (like a written-down body scan). Have a conversation between you and an imaginary person, or between two characters in a story, or between your left foot and your right foot, or between you and your 90-year-old self, or . . .

The potential for dialogue is bottomless. What will your characters talk about? Experiment with very few words, then whole scenes filled with monologues. This is micro-playwriting at its best. If you're feeling brave, get someone to act out the dialogue with you. Is the dialogue natural? Is it true to what that character would say? Here we're working with the relation between speech and writing. Listen out for conversations you hear all around you and use turns of phrase that interest you naturally in your mindful journal.

11 Write a list of nouns

This is a great exercise which we're borrowing from the lovely writer and imagination executive Ray Bradbury. It's really simple and can help in flustered moments where you just don't know where to start and sentences seem too big. Simply put: do a quiet meditation, then gently write a long list of nouns that are in your head. Get the nouns out and on to the page. Write them in capitals, write them really small: however you like them, free these nouns that – somehow – relate to you in this mindful moment.

12 Write letters to your selves

Getting post is one of the best things in life. So to make sure you get some, write a letter to your various selves. It's really easy (though you might need a friend's help).

Do it as you would write a normal letter. Address yourself (use a nickname if you like). Date it. Write about whatever you like but focus on your feelings, any bodily sensations, any plans, dreams or intentions, and always end with a P.S. I call that the P.S. de resistance.

Mix things up a bit: write to your 16-year-old self, or your 66-year-old self (choose ages you're far away from) or a particular body part. What would you tell your younger self? What would you like your older self to have done? What would you say in a letter to your feet?

Now, here's the fun bit. Pop your letter in an envelope, address it to yourself and stamp it, and give it to a friend. Ask them to send it to you when you least expect it. Make sure it's at least six months from now and hopefully longer, so you're really not thinking about it. I guarantee, whenever your friend sends it, it will be relevant to you the day you eventually read it.

13 Write with subtlety

It's crucial to slow down – we know this – to become mindful and to write your journal entries in a mindful way. But it might not be clear why it's crucial. Slowing down to mindful journal time means you get to observe the finer, more subtle side to life. If someone asked you how you were, you might say, 'Oh, I'm fine.' But what if you were in tune with the subtlety of your lived experience in that moment? For instance, you might say something like this in answer to the question, 'How are you?': 'I'm experiencing the subtle playfulness of light and shadow through the window there, and the light has softened my sitting in this moment, so that my shoulders feel lighter, less taut . . .' Of course, we don't speak like that in everyday life (perhaps we're thankful about that), but it doesn't mean we can't in our mindful journals.

Imagine how grateful your much older self will be when he or she reads about your past experience with that level of subtlety and detail. Use variations here to help you get to the subtlety – vary the point of view, vary the angle of approach in your writing, change who's speaking or the focus of your interest. Find the subtlety below the subtlety, and keep going – subtlety is infinite. The great news is, this is further proof there's no such thing as writer's block. Behind every sentence you write there are at least a hundred others.

14 Write about the quality of light

I had an inkling for this workshop idea and then it was all confirmed when I read Pat Schneider's extraordinary book, *How the Light Gets In*. Pat uses a similar exercise in her own workshops. It's a really simple way into writing your mindful journal:

- Meditate on something you are going to write about.
- Find whatever it is, and then ask yourself this one simple question: 'What is the quality of the light in this moment/scene/situation?'
- Write about the quality of the light.

See what happens. What words have you used? Where was the scene? How does writing about the quality of the light affect your understanding of the scene and your writing? What are we talking about when we talk about light? What other kinds of light can you write about? How subtle can you be with your description of the light?

15 Write using the steppingstones method

Ira Progoff's fantastic Intensive Journal Method certainly has bits we can use as mindful journal writers. Steppingstones (I like that it's one long word) helps you uncover any threads or movements in your life. It's a great technique if you're looking for change at the moment, as you can find your personal 'lines of continuity', while you are also generating loads of material to use for future writing. Essentially, using steppingstones involves listing key moments in your life that relate to a theme of your choosing. The generation of the list becomes a fantastic resource you can play with.

Here's how it works. Write eight to twelve steppingstones. These can be key moments in your life, or events, images, sensations or thoughts that relate to a theme. So if, say, 'Body' is your theme, write eight to twelve moments from your life when your body was of interest to you. For example, I'd have these as some of my steppingstones relating to 'Body':

- That time I ran through the playground at primary school and noticed for the first time I had knees.
- When I moved to London on the Sunday and was admitted to hospital on

the Wednesday; face down, my head over the edge of the hospital bed, watching my tears form a pool on the floor.

- That time I fell down to the ground – quite fantastically, my right foot tripped up on my left foot – in front of 30 new colleagues.
- Drinking fizzy water for the first time in my life, one really hot summer as a kid, and loving the way it quenched my thirst.
- My experience of the panic in my own body as a fellow passenger had an epileptic fit on the Underground.

And so on. Don't worry about chronology. You can rearrange the order later. For now, just write eight to twelve steppingstones, according to your chosen theme.

Once you've done this, you'll realize you have some fantastic raw material to work with and on. These moments will come back into your journal, consciously or otherwise, or you can return to this entry and pick different steppingstones as launch pads for future writing. Change the theme of your steppingstones. Here are some to get you started: Work, Life, Love, Childhood, Growing Up, Transitions, Key People, Body Parts, Books, Light . . . Come back to steppingstones practice every so often, even with the same theme. You'll find you have hundreds of steppingstones. They're deep within you.

16 Write borrowing opening lines from great poets

You might have realized by now that I do not believe in the thing some people call 'writer's block'. There are plenty of other things we could be doing in this moment, yes, but writing is always an option. I do have some sympathy though, when it's late and you're tired and you want to write but you don't know what to write about.

So, go fishing. Grab a book from the shelf, open it at a random page and pick a line. There you go, you've just got your first line. Write it out and simply keep on writing. Going fishing applies to lots of things. During the day, jot down any overheard sentences on the bus or that you hear at work by the photocopier. Watch a film with pen and paper at hand and write down any lines of dialogue you love. As a mindful journal writer, you open your heart to what's possible. Go fishing any time.

And especially: fish inwards – note any funny lines in your head, the bits of us that don't come out as speech, that somehow just stay up there. Find yourself, everyone and everything, fascinating. As Theodore Roethke said, live in 'perpetual, great astonishment'. Enjoy fishing and filling up your journal with the world's words.

17 Write with Focusing

Focusing – with a capital F – was discovered (or invented, I'm not sure which) by psychotherapist and philosopher Eugene Gendlin. I've found it to be so useful and beneficial to my mindful journal practice. It looks a bit like mindfulness meditation, but it's got a much more practical, verbal application.

Focusing involves recognizing something inside us Gendlin called the 'felt sense'. If emotions are really obvious instances of affectedness (just look at that angry man over there), and if feelings are clear but often quieter instances of affectedness (I feel sad but I'm not communicating to anyone), the felt sense is the thing that's fuzzy and underneath it all: it's the blurry, unclear, murky quality of our lived experience. Gendlin uses the example of someone going on an aeroplane and having a 'niggling' feeling that they've forgotten to do something. That niggling is a felt sense. I see the felt sense as our lack of clarity, our inarticulacy, which is close to being put into words. In other words, our felt sense is our being about to verbalize something, rooted in our embodiment. So it's ripe for mindful journal practice.

Here's a really easy way to have a go at finding your felt sense and using Focusing to write your mindful journal entries. I've adapted it from Sonia Perls's own writing with Focusing instructions:

- Get comfy in your chair with your mindful journal out in front of you. Close your eyes if you'd like to. Find a way to be quietly and comfortably aware of your inner state.
- Ask yourself, 'How am I in this moment?' Take a minute to jot down a list of answers to this question today.
- Now ask yourself, 'What's up with me today? Of all the things I know about, what might I like to write about in this moment?' Write down what comes. You might get one thing, you might get several things. Even if you write 'Nothing', ask yourself, 'Now what's all this "Nothing" about, hey?'

- Ask yourself, 'Now that I have these words written down, have I missed any out? Could I add just a few more words that help me in this moment with what I want to write about?' Jot them as they come.

- Ask yourself, 'What am I drawn towards from this list of words?' Write the word or idea at the top of a new page in your journal.

- Now, take a deep breath and do some free writing on this topic. Write for at least eight minutes or however long feels good for you in this moment.

- Stop yourself and look over what you've just done. Ask yourself, 'What haven't I said yet? What's at the heart of this issue?' Wait quietly for a word, image or phrase to arise from your felt sense of the topic. Write whatever comes.

- Take this word or image and use it. Ask yourself, 'So what's here?' Describe the feeling, image or word. Let your felt sense deepen. Where do you feel it? In your belly? In your chest? In your neck? Continue to ask yourself, 'Do these words match the feeling? Am I saying it?' See if you can feel it so that you naturally say, 'Oh yes, that's it.'

- When you find yourself stopping, ask, 'What haven't I got down on paper yet?' and again look to your felt sense for a word or an image. Write what comes to your body–mind. If you find yourself stopping, ask yourself, 'What am I trying to say?' Write your answer down.

- Once you feel you're near or at the end, ask yourself, 'Does this feel roughly right?' Look to your felt sense for the answer. Again write down whatever answer comes to you. If the answer is 'No', pause and ask yourself, 'What's missing?' and keep writing.

It's almost as if you're two people on a park bench with this exercise. One of you asks questions, the other of you writes down the answers. They (you) then read back what they've written to check it matches the felt experience of the speaker (you). The speaker (you) then says either way whether it matches your lived experience, and you both continue.

This is a fantastic trick for writing, because it's got an inbuilt Writing Encouragement Mechanism while at the same time offering a way to help match words to the richness and complexity of your lived experience. Focusing is great for helping you deal with your feelings and especially for helping with decision making and moving forward in life.

18 Write your famous last words

Think about your last day on Planet Earth. What would you like your famous last words to be? Write a list of your potential final sentences. Practise saying them. Vary them. Bring attention to your body as you consider them.

19 Write about objects in front of you

This is a really handy exercise if you're a bit stumped today and fancy writing something quite quickly.

- Look around your room. Pick five to ten objects. They don't all need to be too meaningful, though do bung in a couple that really have some personal value to you.
- Lay them out on your writing table, almost the way a still life painter might arrange them.
- Now write your mindful journal with little headings for each object. Describe the object and its meaning to you in this moment. If you've got a music CD there, why that one, why now? What's your relationship with music in your life? If you've got a candle, who gave it to you? How much has burned away? What kinds of conversations have you had around it? Find the questions with the objects.
- Give each item your attention, tell your journal more about it and its meaning to you, and you'll find you have a rather beautiful piece of writing that will surprise you and, in the future, illuminate themes and threads in your life that reappear again and again. After all, you might think you chose those items randomly, but did you, really?

20 Write out your loving-kindness meditation

At the heart of mindfulness meditation is loving-kindness and the intention to work on our very own ability to be loving and kind in our everyday lives, both to ourselves and to others around us. Meditating is itself an act of loving-kindness, as is keeping a mindful journal or walking mindfully. The loving-kindness meditation taught by teachers like Jon Kabat-Zinn involves imagining the love of someone who truly has loved you, and using it to then help you reflect on your love for yourself as well as others (even people you find difficult to love).

There's lots to be said here – we could fill another book – but let's just go straight to the journal writing exercise, because it's a good one:

- Bring to mind someone who you know just loves you. It might be a parent, a partner, a friend, an animal – someone who has unconditional love for you in every respect. If there's not someone living now, think of someone in the past. If no-one comes to mind in this moment, don't worry – just imagine a great unconditional loving directed towards you.

- Now, keeping that person's love for you in your heart, holding it in your body, letting the light of his or her love fall through you, redirect it so that you become both its source and its intended recipient. In other words, send that brilliant loving-kindness to yourself, from yourself.

- As you do so, write these words in your journal (bringing attention to the act of writing as you do):

  May I be safe and protected.
  May I be happy and contented.
  May I be whole and healthy.
  May I experience ease.

- Reread the words you have written down. Feel them. Get underneath them. Lie in them like a comfortable bed with your favourite duvet on Saturday morning.

Do this every day, or any day, or once a year, and vary it: send love out to other people, to animals and indeed to the whole planet. Always start by invoking that great love for you that then turns into love for yourself, but from there you can go anywhere: send love to friends, family members, partners, people you don't know, people you have difficulty with, writers you love, writers you loathe, politicians, peace campaigners, animals, forests, the air, your skin, the planet we live in, the multiverse, a single atom . . . You'll just need to change the words: 'May he be safe . . .', 'May the planet be happy . . .' and so on. This is a great exercise to do when you're feeling a bit tired and can't write much, because the words are already here for you.

21 Write a story about your breath

Here's how. Write about yourself and your day, using quite simple language and in the third person. This is good practice for shifting perspective, step-ping back and having a narrator's view on your own life. Mine might start, for example: 'Philip got up. He seemed quite confused, but he often is when he first wakes up. Philip got out of bed and rubbed his eyes. He walked to the bathroom . . .' Do this for a page or so. Really get into your day. Add some details. Be specific. Feel your hand moving across the page. Then come to a stop whenever you're ready to.

Go back and rub out your name or cross a line through it each time, and change it for 'The breath' or 'Breathing' or simply 'Breath'. Breath is now the character of a short story. Read it out loud. Feel your breathing as you read. 'Breathing got up. He seemed quite confused, but he often is when he first wakes up. Breathing got out of bed and rubbed his eyes. He walked to the bathroom . . .' See where you go with it. After all, it's true, isn't it, that your breath is a leading character in your life?

22 Write about your virtues or values

One of my favourite facts about Benjamin Franklin – founding father of the United States, polymath, inventor of the lightning rod – is that he kept a mindful journal. Well, in a way. Franklin, aged 20, developed a list of 13 virtues that he wanted to live his life by. He wrote them down and each week chose a virtue to practise that week. His virtues included things like Justice, Chastity, Sincerity and Humility. The key thing is that he wrote them down each week and reflected on them, and in his autobiography he wrote, 'I hope that some of my descendants may follow the example and reap the benefit.'

Let's be those descendants and reap the benefit. What are your virtues? Write down a handful in your mindful journal – it needn't be as many as 13! – and describe each one. What virtues do you have which you are clearly aware of? What virtues or values might you have which you aren't so aware of? Perhaps you didn't realize how generous you are? Use this exercise to bring some kind awareness to your kindness and other virtues. For each virtue, write about how you live up to it, add instances in your day that might test your virtue, and so on. If you fancy some inspiration, here are a list of virtues and values you might find useful to write about – and I'm indebted to Kelly McGonigal's work for this exercise (more on her later): Acceptance, Accountability, Art, Celebration, Collaboration, Commitment, Compassion, Competence, Courage, Creativity, Curiosity, Discipline, Discovery, Efficiency,

Equality, Excellence, Fairness, Faith, Freedom, Grace, Gratitude, Happiness, Health, Helping Others, Independence, Integrity, Joy, Leadership, Lifelong Learning, Love, Mindfulness, Nature, Openness, Patience, Pets, Politics, Practical Action, Resourcefulness, Self-reliance, Simplicity, Strength, Tradition, Trust, Willingness, Wisdom. How you relate to each of these values will take a lifetime of journals to fill!

23 Write using bibliomancy

Bibliomancy is a kind of divination by books (it's an ancient Persian practice) and requires a certain amount of gravity, so now's as good a time as any to get bibliomancing. Here's how to give it a try.

Stand next to a bookshelf. Close your eyes and think of a problem or situation going on in your life right now. With your eyes still shut, pass your right or left hand along the shelf until you naturally stop at a book. Pull the book out (keeping your eyes shut). Feel its gravitational pull. Hold it in your hands with your eyes shut. Keep your problem or situation in mind. Flick through the book for a while, as you bring to mind this problem or obstacle or opportunity.

When you are ready, pick a page (your eyes are still shut) and open it. With a finger, and your eyes still shut, keep your situation in mind and find your finger naturally stopping at a certain point on the page. Bring awareness to gravity's pull as you do this.

When your finger has stopped on the page, open your eyes and read the nearest full line or word. Write it down in your journal and either continue writing from that line or just leave it at that today. Did the passage talk to your problem or opportunity? Feel free to give the experiment another try.

24 Write in front of a mirror

Place a mirror in front of yourself – straight on, to the side, however you like – and write in your journal. Every so often, you might look up and notice your reflection, and smile. Or as you're writing, you might extend your attention outwards – not changing the focus of your gaze – so that you can see yourself writing in the perimeter of your looking. Notice the difference between writing with and writing without a mirror. If you can, look up every so often and say, 'You are writing' or 'I love you' to your reflection. Self-love is an integral part of mindfulness and of mindful journalling and this practice really brings that idea home.

25 Write using Sei Shōnagon's lists

I can't recommend reading Sei Shōnagon's court diary, *The Pillow Book,* enough, and one exercise she uses, which could be useful, is writing lists of things. So for this exercise, write lists like Sei Shōnagon, and feel connected to over a thousand years of breathing in between you and her. Here are some list titles to get you started, courtesy of Sei Shōnagon:

- Things that make one's heart beat faster
- Infuriating things
- Elegant things
- Things that arouse a fond memory of the past
- Things that cannot be compared
- Things that have lost their power
- Awkward things
- Things that are distant though near
- Things that should be large
- Things that make the heart lurch with anxiety
- Features I particularly like.

26 Write using double-entry journalling

Quite simply, this is where you give yourself two pages per day, a left page and a right page. You write your journal entry on the right-hand side, say, jotting down whatever you feel like jotting down. Then, over time, you reread your journal entries and use the blank left-hand-side pages to write journal entries about your right-hand-side journal entries. They might focus on patterns spotted, previously unseen, or how the body feels rereading what's been written before. You can also use double-entry journalling on the same day – so write on the right-hand-side first, then reflect on the left – or you can leave a period of time between the two acts of pen pushing.

27 Write what you hear

Here's a really nice exercise to get you writing without thinking. Sit comfortably with your mindful journal in front of you. Close your eyes and bring awareness to what you can hear. Allow sounds to just be. Don't follow them or build up any big stories around them. Just let sounds be. After a good few minutes or so (however long works for you), start writing about what you heard. Use words to capture the quality of the sounds in your soundscape. Use plain language or flowery, metaphor-filled language (however you like). You could list each sound a bit like this: 'Sound of car horn. Sound of door closing. Sound of phone ringing. Sound of man shouting.'

After you've done that, spend some time writing about the sounds of things you didn't hear. For example, the sound of ink drying on the page, the sound of the butterfly landing, the sound inside your socks. I wonder if there is an infinity of sounds we can't hear? Once you've written about both sounds you heard and didn't hear, read back your mindful journal entry, noticing how you sit and breathe in this moment.

28 Write sentences that begin with 'Hello'

Grab your journal, whatever form it takes. I want you to write ten sentences which each begin 'Hello'. With each sentence, I want you to say what you're saying hello to (I'm assuming these will be things you don't normally say hello to). Start with obvious things – 'Hello, my lovely tablecloth' – and then move towards less obvious things – 'Hello, the view out of my window'. You could hello things on your mind – 'Hello, my worry about my friend' – and things that are definitely not here – 'Hello, the UN building' – as well as abstract concepts – 'Hello, freedom' – and any intentions today – 'Hello, my writing 1,000 words by midday'. Say hello to as many things as you like (ten is a good starter). Underline lines that intrigue you about yourself today. Work with those today; make one of them a title and start writing from that. Don't forget to hello yourself, too, even if it's just quietly, under your breath. Finally, feel free to change hello to 'Good morning' or 'Good afternoon' or even 'Hi there' or your preferred salutation. And continue with your regular mindful journal practice from here, closing it with some 'Goodbye' sentences, if that works for you.

29 Write about three different kinds of experience

This is a great exercise to greet the day with, and useful if you're stumped over what to write. Imagine there are three realms or worlds – the outer realm, the inner realm and the realm between. The outer world is anything you can see right now. It can also be things you know to exist but can't see (e.g. the Himalayas). The inner world is any bodily sensation you're experiencing in this moment, or a thought, or anything you're imagining, or a plan, and so on. The realm between is the skin of your body: just notice any sensations on your skin, the bit of you that seems to sum up that betweenness between the outer and the inner world.

For your mindful journal, it's nice to write what you notice in each realm. Write a list-based entry today where each sentence begins 'I notice . . .' Let's notice three things in each realm for now but feel free to go for it if you're on top noticing form today or to spend your whole time focusing on one realm. What do you notice in each of the three realms today, and how do you relate to them?

30 Write with your eyes shut

This is a good one for bringing attention to the relationship between your eyes and the page as you write. Grab your journal and open to an empty page. Notice the size, the edges, the quality of the paper, the light falling on it, your feelings in this moment and anything else that comes up for you. Now get ready to write – and shut your eyes. Write for eight minutes with your eyes shut the whole time. Yes! With eyes shut! Once time's up, read back what you've written. Notice your handwriting, if it's different. Underline words and sentences that surprised you. Carry on writing, eyes opened, if now's good, inspired by writing in the dark like that.

And while you're here: try a similar experiment, but this time write with your non-dominant hand. So if you're right-handed, write with your left hand (and the other way round, obviously). Ambidextrous? Write both ways and record the difference (do you find you've still got a slightly more dominant hand?). Write for eight minutes with your non-dominant hand. Read back what you write. Underline interesting words and phrases. Store these for later or carry on writing now with either hand. Give yourself a round of applause (can you try clapping with just one of your hands?).

Before we stop writing and start reflecting . . .

We're going to move to the next chapter shortly, so it's a good time to reflect on where we are. We've prepared ourselves to write, and we've now written. All that remains is to reflect on our writing – to wonder – and we've got what I'm calling a mindful journal practice. It's writing, knowing it's writing. *Writing, being the knowing that's writing.* Before we do move on, though, I wanted you to try one more kind of mindful journalling. It involves writing a journal entry without writing anything down.

---

31 Write without writing

Imagine opening your journal. Imagine picking up your pen. Then imagine writing a sentence. How does the sentence appear to you in your body-mind? Can you 'write' another one? How does it look on your imaginary page? What's the difference between writing in the 'real world' and writing in your imagination like this? Is there any at all? One philosophical theory – Extended Mind Thesis – suggests there is no difference, in fact. The writing and the imagined writing are both tokens of the same thing. This theory implies that our minds are extended out into the world around us, they're not just bunged up inside our heads. Your mindful journal, then, becomes a part of you, a part of your mind, your extended mind into the world. It's as exciting as that. Take some time with this one. Really be with the imaginary writing. When you're ready, pick up your actual pen and journal and write for real, documenting the difference between the lived sensations of both.

5

Wondering – reflecting on your mindful journal

Pen down (mindfully)

There! You've done it. You've written mindfully in your journal. Your pen's beside your shut journal. You're sitting in the quietness that follows. You're in the aftermath. Aftermath's a lovely word here: it refers to the second going over the mown lawn with the lawnmower, that second wave of cutting grass, that's not so much cutting grass as reflecting on cutting grass.

So just sitting in the silence after writing. Sitting in your sitting. You might just take a moment to sit mindfully, bringing attention to the contact your body makes with the floor and your seat. You might bring awareness to sounds and sights, not following anything, instead just noticing and, if need be, labelling your experiences in your head: *Hearing, hearing, seeing, seeing, feeling, feeling*. Finally, sitting into presence, your presence: presencing, *presence-sing* (as Jon Kabat-Zinn says).

Then, go

It's really important, after writing your mindful journal entries, after a brief moment of mindful pause, to stand up and go. Leave the wooden hut of your awareness. Go and do something else. Your mindful journal is always there for you.

We accept what is here

Whatever it is you have written in your journal, it's really important that you practise accepting it for what it is. So here, we're just letting be what needs to be. We're accepting our words and ourselves for who they and we are. In the classic mindfulness formulation, we're not wanting to change anything, we're just noticing what turns up. So when you put down your pen, you don't rush back in and edit, or scrutinize what you've read, or judge yourself. You practise acceptance – one of the key mindfulness foundations. That means accepting the words, the content of the words, your handwriting, the shape of the words on your page, the number of times you crossed out words, the aesthetics of the page and your journal, how you were feeling while you wrote the words, how you feel about who wrote the words and so on. In fact, the act of writing words down is itself an act of acceptance, so you've already done the hard work.

Accept yourself into existence

On reading back your journal entries, accept yourself so much that you blush, or cry, or laugh. Rather like loving-kindness, acceptance is something like the feeling a grandparent has for a grandchild. While parents might scold their child (thereby judging), grandparents – in that special position of not being the parent – can accept their grandchild more. There's a wisdom, isn't there, in that relationship between grandparent and grandchild, a kind of knowing nod. Tove Jansson's *The Summer Book* – which in its own way reads like a mindful journal – is a good example of this relationship. Can you bring into yourself that knowing, accepting relationship between grandparent and grandchild, as you reflect on your mindful journal entries with loving-kindness?

Write about funny things from your day

I flew to India recently and at the security gate a sign read: 'In case of emergency, you may be required to do a body scan.' I chuckled and thought my fellow mindfulness practitioners would, too.

> Got any jokes? Write them down. It's lovely to see jokes written down on the page. And while you're at it, write down any laughter-based steppingstones in your life. Laughter, and memories of laughter, can encourage even more laughter – and laughter has billions of benefits.
>
> And while you're at it, how about laughing at nothing? Can you practise a bit of laughter yoga in this moment? Just start softly and slowly laughing, no jokes needed, shuffling your shoulders forwards and giving your best chuckles. It really is lovely to fill your mindful journal with laughter. Even when difficulties arise, can you bring some laughter in?

Acceptance is the thing

When we accept how we are in ourselves, we can use the magnifying glass of our heart to zoom up close and personal. Acceptance leads to detail, leads to writing – and detailed acceptance of inner experience from every angle is the key. When we finish our writing, acceptance helps us read back our words with loving, living kindness.

Accepting is both the hardest and the easiest foundational attitude of mindfulness and mindful journal practice. You don't have to do anything other than accept how things are in this moment. It doesn't get more tragic and funny than that.

But a quick note: accepting isn't the same thing as 'putting up with'. Paradoxically, only when you accept who you are can you change. This is like what scientist and judo black belt Moshe Feldenkrais said: 'When you know what you're doing, then you can do what you want.' So reflect on your mindful journal entries with an acceptance that is critically engaged with the whole process, not a lazy acceptance or a reluctant acceptance. Or at least, if it is lazy or reluctant, fully turn up to what it means to be lazy, what it means to be reluctant. If lazy, *be* the laziness.

Vary how you read back your journal entries

Remember how varying things is good for the prone-to-pruning brain? Bring variations into how you read back your journal, as well as how you write it. Can you vary the angle of your eyes in relationship with the page? Move your eyes closer, move them further away. Turn your journal around like a clock and keep trying to read your writing, no matter whether your words are upside down or skew-whiff. It's amazing how you can still read and understand your words, even if they're upside down. Vary where you read your journal, the room, the time of day; vary what you notice (the quality of the paper, the light, the ink). Variations are good not only for your brain but also for your writing; change how you read and I reckon you'll change how you write.

Read your mindful journal in all sorts of bodily positions

Try something different today: read back your mindful journal in different positions. Start reading your journal sitting down. Then stand up and read your journal standing up. Then walk slowly and read your journal walking slowly. Then stop and read your journal standing up again. Then walk slowly back to your chair and read your journal walking slowly back to your chair. Then sit down and read your journal sitting down. Do this as slowly and as lazily as possible, with quick-witted attention to your body and breath in each moment.

Have a go at practising letting go

Letting go and letting be (accepting) go hand in hand. To let something be, to accept it, is to let it go. Letting go – or non-attachment – is
achieving a black belt in the karate of now. Noticing how you attach
yourself to various things on the planet – material objects, people,
ideas – and how you then detach yourself is one of the most fascinating, continuing aspects of living what Jon Kabat-Zinn calls 'the full
catastrophe'. To use the karate metaphor again, letting go is that final
chop through wood. Between the moment the hand finishes touching
the wood to the moment the hand is free from it, that's letting go.

In other words, when you stop writing and come towards your
mindful journal with an attitude of quiet reflection, try and inhabit
the foundational attitude of letting go. Be ready to look at your words
in order to let go of them. Think of your reading as a kind of letting
go. You're looking at words to let go of them. It's as though you want
to hold hands because you love letting go of them so much.

Reflect on why you're doing this again

It's worth having a quick look back at your great expectations and
intentions for this work and in this moment to bring to your heart
the question: 'Why am I keeping a mindful journal at all? What's the
point? Why do all this?' Here's a bit of what I've been suggesting:

- Keeping a mindful journal can form part of a mindfulness meditation practice. It can help you keep meditating regularly and it
  can help you understand what you are doing as you meditate.
  You can bring words to the wordlessness of your body. If you read
  back through your mindful journals over time, you can spot self-
  sequences, which might help you understand yourself more. The
  great Quaker founder, George Fox, invited us all to 'Be patterns' –
  but don't we need help spotting our very own patterns?
- Your journal entries are also reminders of a presence – your presence. They remind you: you were here. We can lose our sense

of connectedness with ourselves – all our selves – but a mindful journal goes some way to recording a connected self. When we die, our mindful journals – if we're happy with them being read by other people – are going to be beautiful, lasting gifts for the recipients of them.

- There is evidence for health benefits from writing like this. I mentioned Dr Pennebaker earlier. In his book, *Opening Up: The healing power of expressing emotions*, Pennebaker explains how self-expression can keep us healthy and well. He carried out experiments with people who had experienced some kind of trauma; they were divided into four groups. Each group wrote for 15 minutes a day for four consecutive days. They were invited to write about different things: the first group wrote about the facts of the trauma; the second group the facts and their emotional responses; a third group only their emotional responses; and the fourth group trivial things like what they had for lunch that day. Following up with the people six months later, Pennebaker found that the second group – those people who had written about both the trauma and their emotional response – had sought medical support 50 per cent less than in the months previous to doing the writing experiment. So the point is: keeping things in can increase your need to seek medical support and expressing things on the page (both the facts and the emotions connected with them) can improve your immune system.

- Other evidence shows that writing about your values can help give your life increased meaning over time. In the 1990s, a group of Stanford students agreed to keep journals over the winter holidays. Some were asked to write about their important values and how their day related to those values. Others were asked to write simply about good things that happened to them. We might say this is the difference between mindful journal writing and normal journal writing. After the break, the students were asked about their holidays. Those who had written about their values were in better health and spirits. They had experienced fewer illnesses and health problems. The reason? The researchers collected all the thousands of journal entries and analysed them: writing about values helped the students see the meaning in their lives. Stressful experiences were no longer hassles; they became an expression of their life values. Writing about your values is the most studied psychological intervention. As psychologist Kelly McGonigal says, 'In the short term, writing about personal values makes people feel more powerful, in control, proud and strong. It also makes them feel more loving, connected, and empathetic towards others. It increases pain tolerance, enhances self-control and reduces unhelpful rumination after a stressful experience.' A meta-study, assessing over 15 years of these sorts of studies, shows that writing about values transforms how you think about stressful experiences and your ability to cope with them.

- When you write in your mindful journal you are connecting up to hundreds of thousands of other people who are writing in this moment, trying to capture their experience on the page through words, and with all the many, many more people throughout time who have done the same. As with breathing, our writing practice connects us up to the wholeness of humanity. It is our beating heart we are writing and that heart is part of humanity's own vast beating heart. When we write mindfully, our hearts break open with grace, gratitude and gusto. We cannot help but feel effortlessly part of a magnificent wholeness that is both part of us and beyond us at once.

There are lots of things you could do in the moments just after writing in your mindful journal

1 Meditate briefly before carrying on with living. Or perhaps meditating is living for you. Either way is lovely.
2 Stand up straight away and go and do something different.
3 Dance.
4 After a brief moment of pause, rest or meditation, read back what

you've written today; or read back what you've written on other days. What's it like reading these words now?

5 After a brief pause, read back what you've written either today or on other days and then carry on writing. Perhaps what felt like the end was just a temporary end – like most ends – and you were in fact just having a break. It's great to have breaks, I can't recommend them enough in mindful journal practice and life in general.

6 Invite a friendly person to join you and ask him or her to listen as you read out some of your words. (This is a tricky one, as lots of emotions, feelings and bodily sensations may arise in doing this. As long as you don't mind and *do* body, trusting the wisdom of yourself and knowing you can stop reading out loud at any time, you'll be fine. You might ask your friendly person to comment on your words or not, but either way do be clear about that. One lovely thing to ask your friend to do is jot down any phrases he or she particularly liked, but not to interrupt you while you're reading. You can then get your friend to read these out when you finish. It's in its own way quite soothing to do this, and reassuring, and focuses on positivity. After all, this is journalling, you're not submitting a novel to an editor.)

7 Read your words out loud into a voice-recording device or app, then play it back while you are meditating in lying down position. This allows you to let your own words – and voice – sweep and spill all over you and settle into different parts of your body. Using that idea of the felt sense from Focusing, in this way you're checking whether your words match your body's felt sense. It's great, too, because those words were somehow inside you before, but now they are outside you, dancing around your body. It helps you experience being *with* your life, rather than being wrapped up in it. Which words fall where on your body?

8 You could continue writing as a form of reflection. So after closing your journal, you open it again (perhaps changing pens), and this time you write about your recent experience of

mindful journalling. This is a meta-awareness activity, because the chances are you were very aware the first time.

9 Act. Do something. Writing mindfully is really good practice for being. Now you need to practise doing. Feel free to bring mindfulness to the doing, but make sure it's doing you're doing. No *deciding* to do something here please (and then not doing it, if procrastination is one of your hobbies, like mine) – I want proper action. Really enjoy it, especially the difference between doing and the being of your mindful journal practice. What might be the same, though, in each? What thread runs through both being and doing?

10 Make a spaghetti bolognese.

11 Take a rest but then return to your journal and highlight phrases and ideas you like, and which you would like to work on further for published or performed works. You might want to write a poem, or start a short story, or write a play – the ideas for which came about through the act of mindful journalling. So now you're striving – but that's great, because you're not mindful journalling any more. Strive away. The future of the history of literature depends on you. You couldn't have got to that poem without the mindful journalling, and vice versa.

A quick reminder of what we've been up to

With mindful journal practice, you do three things:

- Gathering – the first thing you do is stop, slow down and prepare to write in your journal.
- Jotting – the second thing you do is write in your journal.
- Wondering – and the third thing you do is reflect – in some way – on what's just happened.

We do all three parts with mindfulness (non-judgemental moment-to-moment awareness) and it can take any amount of clock time – from five minutes to a whole afternoon or day – because it's all unfolding in the great long now. With mindful journal practice, you tell yourself – and the universe – your story. This is the account of your hut, don't forget. It's as simple, and difficult, as that.

Afterword

Your journal – the mindful hitchhiker's guide to the galaxy

Afterword, afterwards, after words

I, like you, like words. I like the word 'afterword', which is often the writer's closing thoughts, or after thoughts, at the end of a book. After all, there's a sense here of being after something, the opposite of forwards, foreword, for words. We're at the end of something. With mindfulness, of course, all endings are only ever temporary.

I like the way 'after words' has two distinct meanings: the sense of being after or behind or at the end of something, and the second meaning of the sense of longing for something. Mindfulness practice is founded on this question: what do you long for? What words are you after? With mindful journalling, we are literally after words: we are gently trying to find the words to name our experience, to bring experience to light but also to name the darkness that the light is premised on. Once we have written in our journals, we sit in the experience after words.

In a way, of course, your mindful journal will never come to an end

Unlike this book, your journal lives on and on and on. It will live as long as you live, in all its various forms and guises. And even when you die, won't something of it still live on? Isn't there something shared in all this inner and outer experience? So that when we die our mindful journals simply pass on to the next investigative journalist of the heart in a way: which is a reminder that our own mindful journals are a continuation of an enduring bewilderment and astonishment about lived experience – we pick up where others left off. In a funny way, our mindful journals are not so much about us as such, but about experience and the experience of experience.

I have various images of you in my head as we come to a close

You are wild journal keeper, mindful journal practitioner, investigative journalist of the heart, scribbler down of wonder. And in this moment I have a gentle image in my head of you putting your journal and pen away and standing up and walking off.

It is important to walk away, isn't it, and you're doing that right now. You almost look like a shepherd. It's almost as if we're out on some plain somewhere, or on some hills. Yes, let's pretend we're on a vast hill or plain, and you're a shepherd, and there are thousands of stars up above. It is dusk. You've just stood up, having done some writing in your journal, and you're now heading off. Indeed, your whole body is heading off, not just your head. You turn around briefly (what turns first?), you give me a kind and knowing nod (I'm smiling too) and then you saunter off, your pockets full of party-poppers, ready to celebrate each moment.

Saunter is such a great word for walking in a certain way

This is definitely the kind of walking a mindful journal keeper would do. You're one of those 'one or two persons' whom Thoreau describes in his essay 'Walking' as having 'a genius, so to speak, for sauntering'. Wondering about the origin of the word 'saunter', he suggests it comes from one of two things: either it refers to those holy people who walked to the Holy Land – *à la sainte terre* – or it refers to those people who are *sans terre*, literally without a home, the homeless (those who can but saunter).

I think this mindful journal malarkey involves a kind of sauntering of sorts (a kind of holiness, a kind of homelessness), except the landscape isn't just out there (it very much is out there) so much as it's in here, across the way, behind the back, through the middle, upside down . . .

When we keep a mindful journal, we saunter in every direction of ourselves. In a way, we saunter through the universe, like Douglas Adams's famous hitchhiker, taking note of what we see and feel and think and embody, of who we are, of who we are becoming. With mindful journal practice, we investigate our sense of self and the sensing of our physical self – our continuities and our newfangledness.

To write mindfully about the present moment connects us up, somehow, with a universe that is not only invested in this idea of being connected up but ultimately reliant on it. Describe doing the dishes and you've probably written a poem about Jupiter.

You're doing brilliantly

Keep going. Write wonderful things. Be braver than you can be, and more generous than you thought possible. Dish the muck, polish the silver. Go up close to as much or as little as you fancy. To misquote Baloo the bear from the film *The Jungle Book*: fall apart in your own back yard.

And do keep in touch – let me know how your mindful journalling goes. Keeping in touch, in fact, is the thing. That's what we're doing with mindful journalling: we're keeping in touch: with ourselves, with each other, with the universe, with our beautiful, beating – wild, flapping – hearts.

Before you go: one last exercise

Here's a question for you. I'd like to whisper it in your ear but I'd also like you to write it in your journal in a whispery kind of way. So whisper-write the following question at the top of your next blank page in your journal and just see how it lands. Feel free to answer it or just let it settle in your body as you gently come back to look at it:

Aren't you writing your mindful journal because you've come back to your life and you're a little bit – even just a little bit – more in love?

One last thing: mindful journalling is all about saving the day

I mean this in the sense that, with this work, you are storing the day, keeping it – or something of it, at least – for yourself, for others, for life. I also mean that mindful journalling is somehow about healing or solving the day, finding some kind of salvation for it, or indeed searching for an answer to that tricky question the poet Philip Larkin famously posed, and which can still elude even the best of ourselves: what are days for?

My suggestion to you, as you slowly begin to put this book down now and start to pick up your pen of beginner's mind and hand, is that you journal mindfully when you realize that – to coin a phrase – only *you* can save the day.

Further reading

Anat Baniel, *Move into Life: The nine essentials for lifelong vitality*, New York: Random House (2009)

Elisabeth Bishop, *One Art: The selected letters*, London: Pimlico (1996)

Bok, *Words Out of Silence: 60 days in solitude*, California: Non-Duality Press (2014)

Ray Bradbury, *Zen in the Art of Writing: Essays in creativity*, New York: Bantam (1920, third edition 1994)

Joe Brainard, *I Remember*, New York: Granary Books (2001)

Peter Elbow, *Everyone Can Write: Essays toward a hopeful theory of writing and teaching writing*, Oxford: Oxford University Press (2000)

Christopher Germer, *The Mindful Path to Self-Compassion*, New York: The Guilford Press (2009)

Natalie Goldberg, *Writing Down the Bones: Freeing the writer within*, Boston, Massachusetts: Shambhala Publications (2005)

Burghild Nina Holzer, *Walk Between Heaven and Earth: A personal journal on writing and the creative process*, New York: Random House USA (1994)

Tove Jansson, *The Summer Book*, London: Sort Of Books (2003)

Derek Jarman, *Modern Nature: The journals of Derek Jarman*, London: Vintage (1992)

Jon Kabat-Zinn, *Coming to our Senses: Healing ourselves and the world through mindfulness*, London: Piatkus (2005)

Jon Kabat-Zinn, *Full Catastrophe Living: How to cope with stress, pain and illness using mindfulness meditation*, London: Piatkus (revised edition 2013)

David McCown and Marc S. Micozzi, *New World Mindfulness: From the founding fathers, Emerson, and Thoreau to your personal practice*, Randolph, Vermont: Healing Arts Press (2012)

Kelly McGonigal, *The Upside of Stress: Why stress is good for you and how to get good at it*, New York: Avery (2015)

Sarah Manguso, *Ongoingness: The end of a diary*, Minneapolis, Minnesota: Graywolf Press (2015)

Thich Nhat Hanh, *The Miracle of Mindfulness: The classic guide to meditation by the world's most revered master*, London: Rider (2008)

Solomon Northup, *Twelve Years a Slave: A true story*, London: Collins (2014)

Ben Okri, *A Time for New Dreams*, London: Rider (2011)

Mary Oliver, *Long Life: Essays and other writing*, Boston, Massachusetts: Da Capo (2004)

Parker J. Palmer, *A Hidden Wholeness: The journey toward an undivided life*, San Francisco: Jossey-Bass (2004)

James Pennebaker, *Opening Up: The healing power of expressing emotions*, New York: Guilford Press (1997)

Fernando Pessoa, *The Book of Disquiet*, London: Penguin (2015)

Ira Progoff, *At a Journal Workshop: Writing to access the power of the unconscious and evoke creative ability*, Los Angeles: Jeremy P. Tarcher (1992)

David K. Reynolds, *Constructive Living*, Honolulu: University of Hawaii Press (1984)

May Sarton, *Journal of a Solitude*, New York: W. W. Norton (1993)

Pat Schneider, *How the Light Gets In: Writing as a spiritual practice*, New York: OUP USA (2013)

Sei Shōnagon *The Pillow Book of Sei Shōnagon*, London: Penguin (1971)

Kate Thompson, *Therapeutic Journal Writing: An introduction for professionals*, London: Jessica Kingsley (2010)